"*People with hidden disabilities have an added handicap—no one can see our pain. The support freely given to those who are ill is often missing when there is no outward sign of disability and we are met instead with disbelief.* Living Well with a Hidden Disability *deals with the physical, emotional, and spiritual facets of invisible illness and teaches you how to cope. It will help enrich your relationships and guide you on a path to healthier living.*"

—Devin J. Starlanyl, former ER physician, now author and president of the Fibromyalgia and Chronic Myofascial Pain Syndrome Institute, Inc.

"*This is a wise, clear book that reveals the practicalities and particulars of how to live more effectively with emotional or physical hidden disabilities. This book is a major contribution to the healing literature on how to change your inner and outer life. A real inspiration!*"

—Diane Shainberg, PhD, author of *Healing in Psychotherapy* and *Path and Process of Inner Change*

"*Stacy Taylor has written a sensitive and informative book. Beginning with her own story, she offers a practical guide for both those who suffer from hidden disabilities and those who want to better understand hidden disabilities. I highly recommend this very readable and caring book.*"

—Melene Smith, MFCC, co-author of *A Women's Midlife Companion: The Essential Resource for Every Woman's Journey*

"*As a nurse and researcher of chronic pain, I have heard many tragic stories like those of Linda, Gina, and Louise, whom you will meet in the pages of this book. Their disability is invisible, their hope fragile, and their suffering profound. I am heartened by this excellent compendium of strategies for self-healing and empowerment. Every individual with a hidden disability can find practical, constructive advice is this book. Their loved ones, doctors, and therapists should read it, too!*"

—Sandra P. Thomas, PhD, RN, FAAN, professor at University of Tennessee at Knoxville and editor of *Issues in Mental Health Nursing*

LIVING WELL WITH A HIDDEN DISABILITY

Transcending Doubt and Shame and Reclaiming Your Life

Stacy Taylor, M.S.W., L.C.S.W.
with Robert Epstein, Ph.D.

New Harbinger Publications

Publisher's Note

This publication is designed to provide accurate and authoritative information in regard to the subject matter covered. It is sold with the understanding that the publisher is not engaged in rendering psychological, financial, legal, or other professional services. If expert assistance or counseling is needed, the services of a competent professional should be sought.

Distributed in the U.S.A. by Publishers Group West; in Canada by Raincoast Books; in Great Britain by Airlift Book Company, Ltd.; in South Africa by Real Books, Ltd.; in Australia by Boobook; and in New Zealand by Tandem Press.

Copyright © 1999 by Stacy Taylor, M.S.W., L.C.S.W., and Robert Epstein, Ph.D.
     New Harbinger Publications, Inc.
     5674 Shattuck Avenue
     Oakland, CA 94609

Cover design © 1999 by Lightbourne Images.
Edited by Angela Watrous.
Text design by Tracy Marie Powell.

Library of Congress Catalog Card Number: 98-68747
ISBN 1-57224-132-2 Paperback

All Rights Reserved

Printed in the United States of America on recycled paper

New Harbinger Publications' Website address: www.newharbinger.com

01 00 99

10 9 8 7 6 5 4 3 2 1

First printing

Dedicated to our parents, Helen and Richard Taylor
and
Evelyn and Harry Epstein, with love and gratitude.

*In the depth of winter I finally learned
that within me there lay an invincible summer.*

—Albert Camus

Contents

First and foremost, I want to thank Robert Epstein, Ph.D., my companion in work and life for the last twenty years. We conceived this book together. His stalwart belief in my ability to write a book sustained me when I had doubts. Robert carefully reviewed and edited each chapter, brainstormed ideas with me, and compiled the list of organizations. On a personal level, I am grateful for his loyalty and devotion during all these years of living with my hidden disability.

Robert and I would like to acknowledge the following people for their interest in this project and their support during the difficult years of coping with chronic pain and illness:

Sheridan Adams, Audrey Adelson, Louise Adler, Sydney Buice, Lucy Childs, Diane Deering-Paulsen, Geri Degen, Dawn Delmonte, Don DiRocco, Debbie Edwards, Martin Epstein, Mark Greenberg, Tom Hendrickson, Ricki Jacobs, Liz Kamens, Jeff Kitzes, Brian Lux, Dan Malcore, Roger Morrison, Ilene Paluck, Sherry Phillips, Penny Pridemore, Judy Rader, Marilee Richards, Jay Schlesinger, Marilyn Schreiber, Melene Smith, Sophie Soltani, Linda Spangler, Cindy Tilton, Miriam Wald, Pam Webb, Liz Weidinger, and Pam Winthers.

We'd also like to thank the staff at New Harbinger Publications for their editorial expertise and enthusiasm for this book.

—Stacy Taylor

Introduction

Stacy Taylor

As a writer and psychotherapist in the San Francisco Bay Area, I specialize in health issues. But my interest isn't strictly professional. Six years ago I developed symptoms of a painful and mysterious disorder that has only intensified while eluding the multitude of medical professionals I've consulted.

I was, at the time, an extremely active and fit thirty-six-year-old. I worked out rigorously three times a week at the gym and devoted weekends to hiking and biking. I took pride in receiving compliments about my muscular physique and stamina. All this changed during an otherwise unremarkable workout at the gym. In a rush to meet a friend, I hopped on a Nautilus adductor machine right after walking on the Stairmaster for thirty minutes, rather than stretching first as usual. My muscles taut from the aerobic workout, I felt a ripping sensation and excruciating pain in my hip. I tried to ignore the pain the first day but then found myself unable to walk. After a few days of taking it easy, I returned to my usual routine of workouts and hiking.

A few weeks later, however, I felt a sharp pain in my lower back when I bent over. Soon thereafter, the pain started spreading—down my leg to my feet and ankles, and into my neck, waxing and waning for no apparent reason. Then even more unusual symptoms appeared, such as tinnitus, vertigo, and rashes. I ran low-grade fevers for no reason. My blood pressure dropped precipitously. I had severe reactions to common medications.

My doctors considered and ruled out a dizzying and frightening array of possibilities, from multiple sclerosis to lupus to cancer. I had innumerable laboratory tests, MRIs, and X rays, all of which were normal. My doctors pronounced me healthy, telling me to go home and deal with my level of stress.

But my major stress was getting sicker with no one knowing why. New symptoms appeared on a weekly basis. I began doctor shopping, seeing more health care professionals than I can even count. I tried various special diets. I gave up sugar, alcohol, caffeine, and white flour. I stayed home, rested, avoided stressful people and situations, and took copious amounts of vitamins and herbs. I meditated, stretched, and practiced positive thinking. All of this experimentation had a major impact on my pocketbook (to the tune of about $7,000) but didn't make a dent in my symptoms.

I received a number of confusing and contradictory diagnoses. A couple of doctors said I had chronic fatigue syndrome, even though I didn't experience severe fatigue or respiratory symptoms. Fibromyalgia was considered but ruled out because I had only one of the eighteen requisite tender points. When a physician diagnosed me with thyroiditis, an autoimmune disorder, I was elated: finally, a diagnosis! But while the thyroid medication helped some symptoms, it worsened others, and I had to stop using it. Candida and food allergies were popular diagnoses, but omitting certain foods had no effect on my symptoms. Probably the most common diagnosis from health care professionals was, "I don't know."

Now, years later, not much has changed for me medically. I still have pretty much the same symptoms; some have gotten worse while others have eased up a bit. I infrequently visit doctors. Occasionally I'll hear of some new treatment and explore it. Unfortunately, I'm generally out a few hundred more dollars with no improvement—and sometimes new side effects from the treatment.

While my physical state has remained the same, developing health problems has changed me enormously. I'm not the same person I was before. There have been enormous losses—of favorite activities and of some friends who lacked understanding. I've shed the illusion that somehow I'm special and can escape the inevitable hardships of a human life—illness, pain, and death.

But the gains have been momentous as well. Learning that life is unpredictable and impermanent has been a gift. I appreciate fully the sacred nature of pain-free moments. I cherish those friends and family members who have remained loving and committed during the rough times. And I no longer discuss pain and grief as an interesting academic discussion topic. I live it. Consequently, I'm a more empathic therapist and a more compassionate human being.

I've also realized firsthand the challenges of living with a hidden disability, which compelled me to write this book. As a traditionally trained therapist, I had adopted the accepted view that illnesses resulted from repressed traumas or depression. The solutions to pain were simple: recall unconscious memories and ventilate feelings. I see now that there are no easy answers to why anyone becomes ill. And making simplistic declarations that illness is due to stress, depression, or bad karma is extremely unfair and often inaccurate.

Just like you, I know how skeptical others can be when your disability is hidden. I've had numerous experiences dealing with people's doubt and ignorance. Fortunately, I've also been moved by those who've been supportive, kind, and understanding. Although I've encountered insensitive health care professionals, I've been grateful for the many who tried their best to help.

This book is the culmination of the lessons I've learned as I struggle to live well with a hidden disability. The book has also been enriched by the courage and tenacity of my clients. The lessons: love yourself no matter how you look or feel. Believe in yourself even if people question your symptoms. Trust that you have the inner strength and perseverance to survive whatever life hands you. Maintain hope that the next day will be easier.

Robert and I, as a couple for over twenty years, have traveled down this difficult path together. We know the impact of a hidden disability on your inner world and family life. In producing this book, we've worked collaboratively; I've been the author, with Robert helping me to brainstorm ideas and polish the text. We offer this book to you in the hopes that you can gain comfort and guidance as you navigate your own journey. You wouldn't have chosen to live with chronic pain, illness, or a psychiatric disability. However, with patience, faith, and fortitude, you can find your way through the dark woods. Your disabilities may or may not be healed physically, but you can become stronger, wiser, and deeper. And maybe this is what defines true healing.

What to Expect from This Book

A few words about how this book is arranged. Part I, "The Experience of Living with a Hidden Disability," covers all aspects of your daily experience. You'll read about the range of common emotions, with numerous suggestions for combating depression and anxiety. We also address the impact on your daily life, including work, love, sex, parenting, and dating.

In Part II, called, "Surviving and Thriving," you'll be offered practical suggestions for rebuilding self-esteem, coping with pain, working with medical professionals and psychotherapists, and nourishing your body and spirit. Since a hidden disability is a family affair, appendix A is written for your loved ones—your partner, friends, family members, or adult children. This appendix is intended to help your loved ones learn ways to support you and themselves. Appendix B offers recommendations for psychotherapists working with clients challenged by hidden disabilities. Appendix C lists helpful books, and appendix D lists national organizations.

While we're confident that this book can help you better cope, it's no substitute for professional advice. If you are seriously depressed and/or suicidal, seek help immediately. If any of the exercises suggested make you feel agitated, discontinue them. You may then choose to reattempt them in a counseling session if so desired.

PART I

The Experience of Living with a Hidden Disability

CHAPTER 1

What Is a Hidden Disability?

Sometimes I wish I looked disabled. Then maybe people could see how much I'm hurting inside.

—Joan, who has chronic
fatigue syndrome

Aimee, age twenty, boards a city bus with her guide dog. She's helped on board by a passenger, and a crowd parts to allow her to sit in the front row. Another passenger admires her dog. When Aimee stands up to leave, two people offer to guide her down the steps and onto the street.

Joan, also twenty, has no obvious disability, but her joints ache and she's exhausted. She takes great care to walk up the steps on the bus, much to the chagrin of impatient passengers. When she finds no seat, she asks a man if she can have his. He ignores her. She stands precariously while holding the handgrip. When the bus arrives at her stop, her slow pace prevents her from making it off the bus in time. She's near tears by the time she gets off at the next stop, several blocks from her intended destination.

These are two disabled people, with very different stories to tell. Aimee's disability was obvious to all around her. People enjoyed helping her. Joan, however, appearing youthful and healthy, elicited a different reaction—impatience, doubt, and neglect. These examples point to the reason why Joan's disability is "hidden." Like Aimee, Joan has more difficulty than the average person when performing small tasks that others can do with ease, like riding a bus. Her physical symptoms disable her. Yet the world doesn't recognize her disability, which makes it hard for Joan to receive needed help or understanding.

While living with any disability is difficult, there are unique challenges when your problems are invisible. Your requests for special needs often evoke skepticism. You may therefore have a harder time asserting yourself and feeling entitled to special help. Many health care professionals question whether your disability is real, especially if no tests confirm it. While a doctor certainly wouldn't dismiss Aimee's vision problems as psychological, you may be told that your pain is "all in your head." Perhaps you're sent to a therapist to deal with underlying conflicts and issues. You start wondering yourself whether you're imagining the whole thing.

Though hidden disabilities are misunderstood, more and more people are stricken with them. The rates of cancer have skyrocketed. The numbers of allergies, neurological diseases, and autoimmune problems have also grown. New and unusual immune disorders have burgeoned. The impact on home, work, and self-esteem is often devastating.

Do You Have a Hidden Disability?

Let's look at what constitutes a hidden disability. We'll then describe the types of hidden disabilities. Also included in this chapter are various theories about what causes these types of disabilities.

Here are the criteria for a disorder to be considered a hidden disability. Your condition should meet most of the following:

1. Impairment in functioning: Your disability reduces your ability to function. An occasional tension headache that's alleviated by aspirin wouldn't apply. Chronic migraines, however, that force you to miss days of work and relentlessly search for a remedy would qualify. You can't work to your normal capacity. Your relationships suffer. Simple chores, such as paying bills or cleaning the bathroom, become monumental.

2. Decrease in quality of life: Your quality of life seriously declines. While once you lived a full life, you're now significantly limited. Your world has become smaller.

3. Restricted lifestyle: You're challenged by your disability daily. Your problems restrict your social and work lives.

4. Focus on pain: You cope with pain, fatigue, and/or discomfort on a regular basis. You may at times feel well but then have flare-ups. Your life is focused on your disability.

5. Feeling defensive: People don't discern that you have a disability. You have to explain or defend your condition to others.

6. Stigma: There's a stigma associated with your disorder. Sometimes people doubt you or trivialize your symptoms. You feel blamed by others for developing a hidden disability.

7. Chronicity: Your disorder is chronic or progressive. Getting a nasty cold a few times a year wouldn't meet this criteria. However, chronic asthma that limits your activities, makes you a frequent visitor to your doctor's office, and causes you to lose work would fit. Occasionally feeling blue wouldn't be a hidden disability. However, chronic depression would apply.

8. Feeling misunderstood: The problem may be misconstrued or misinterpreted. A stroke survivor or a multiple sclerosis sufferer with an unsteady gait may be accused of being drunk. The person with chronic fatigue syndrome who has severe memory loss may be seen as flaky. The pain sufferer who gains weight is perceived as weak and lazy.

Does your health problem meet most of these criteria? If so, you're living with a hidden disability. If your life feels overwhelming, even unmanageable, it's no wonder. You're debilitated by symptoms that are not recognized by the world. You're probably anxious about your future. If your symptoms wax and wane, you feel helpless and out of control. You don't know if your future will bring further deterioration, stabilization, or improvement.

Your life can feel like it's on hold. If you dream of returning to school, you wonder whether you can manage it. Perhaps you long for a child, but you're putting it off until you're better. Or you'd like to buy a house but question whether you can afford the mortgage.

A hidden disability means living with uncertainty. You may search for a doctor who can offer you an answer about why you're sick and how to get better. While many health care professionals try to help, their advice is often contradictory. One doctor says to rest, while another recommends exercise. You may receive various diagnoses. Many clinicians are as puzzled as you about your condition. While a certain medication may be miraculous for a friend, you just get heartburn. Yoga is touted as a pain reliever, but your symptoms become even worse when you try it out. You're left to your own devices to figure out what treatments, if any, work.

This experience of confusion, endless searching outside yourself, and helplessness is typical of living with a hidden disability. While an obvious disability like blindness or paralysis involves a multitude of stresses and adjustments, the condition is generally stable. But with many hidden disabilities, you don't know from one day to the next how you'll feel. New symptoms spring up out of nowhere raising fears of further incapacitation. In the past, when you fell ill with the flu or broke your leg, you had a reasonable idea of when you'd recover. Now you don't know if you'll feel better in two days or two years.

Perhaps you've been a person who's felt in control of your life. You've achieved some status in the world. You've chosen an amiable and compatible mate. You've worked hard all week and had fun on the weekend. A hidden disability turns your life upside down. Nothing feels certain, not even how you'll feel the next day. You may not be able to do something as simple as eating a cookie without exacerbating your problems. A short bike ride may evoke fear of causing a relapse. If your disability is psychiatric, like panic disorder, you also may not even be able to predict a reoccurrence. A panic attack happens out of nowhere—while you're in bed, at a party, on a date. In sum, having any type of hidden disability leaves you feeling frightened, baffled, and out of control.

If you're reading this and nodding your head affirmatively, know that you're not alone. Millions of others are living with a hidden disability. They, too, know the discouragement, fear, and frustration of living with pain and illness that others don't recognize.

While having a hidden disability involves major challenges, it can be handled with dignity and hope. It is possible to live a fulfilling and meaningful life even with physical or emotional disabilities. But it's not easy; it means facing your losses, making adjustments, and developing a realistic attitude. In fact, enduring pain and illness can foster wisdom and compassion. You might not have chosen a hidden disability as your path to deeper maturity, yet your courage and tenacity can inspire others. Throughout this book we'll offer you guidance, suggestions, and emotional support for living well with a hidden disability. Know that you're not alone on this journey.

Types of Hidden Disabilities

While there are commonalties among people with hidden disabilities, there are unique traits as well. We'll next review some of the common types of hidden disabilities, discussing the particular challenges involved in each.

Controversial Diagnoses

When Connie, age thirty-five, saw a new physical therapist for her fibromyalgia (FMS), he declared, "I don't know if FMS is a real problem. I think we have to first get you started on stress management." The physical therapist's reaction was a common one in the life of an FMS sufferer. People with chronic fatigue and immune dysfunction syndrome (CFIDS) and multiple chemical sensitivities (MCS) also face similar skepticism.

Part of the problem is that mostly women fall victims to these disorders. Throughout history, "women's" diseases have been trivialized and psychoanalyzed. Even today, diseases that affect mostly women, such as breast cancer, are routinely underfunded. Premenstrual syndrome (PMS) was for years dismissed as psychological. However, doctors now recognize the pivotal role of hormones in PMS.

Given that strange disorders have cropped up that primarily affect women and have no objective tests to prove them, many health care professionals remain doubtful. When a rash of cases of CFIDS first appeared in Lake Tahoe, Nevada, in 1985, the Centers for Disease Control (CDC) ignored the epidemic for years, claiming CFIDS was a psychosomatic disorder (Johnson 1996). The media gave the illness the pejorative name "yuppie flu." Now the CDC admits that there may be five hundred times as many CFIDS sufferers as it previously estimated. CFIDS has been added to its list of "Priority One New Diseases" (Khalsa 1998).

MCS is another disorder that arouses skepticism. Medical science has a hard time accepting a disorder that's likely caused by the air we breathe and the water we drink. The enormity of the problem of toxic chemicals overwhelms scientists. How do you clear the air of tens of thousands of chemicals used routinely in every segment of society? Rather than condemn society's use of dangerous chemicals, it's easier to dismiss MCS sufferers as emotionally disturbed. Their strange appearance—thin, pale, using gas masks to breathe, and carting along oxygen—attracts stares and smirks. Yet there's an ever-growing number of scientists and health care advocates who take seriously the plight of those with MCS and see all of society at risk.

If you're living with a controversial diagnosis, you're coping regularly with the skepticism of others. But even if your problems defy medical knowledge, this doesn't mean your symptoms aren't real. How the human body functions—and malfunctions—is not totally understood. Scientists are just beginning serious studies to learn how the immune system works.

You also may have a problem that's hard to diagnose. Linda Hanner has written about her six-year journey in search of a cause for her mysterious symptoms. The answer for Hanner was Lyme's disease, an illness that's especially hard to diagnose because of the high rate of false negative blood tests (Hanner 1991). Other cases abound: A thirty-two-year-old woman, Gina, became gravely ill with malnutrition before doctors recognized her disorder as a severe gluten intolerance. An adolescent, Steve, was sent to a psychiatrist to treat personality changes before an MRI revealed a benign, but large, brain tumor.

If you're convinced that your illness is real, just undiagnosed, it takes energy, money, and perseverance to discover your diagnosis. And, for many people, the answer may never be known. Some experts believe that there are new viruses sprouting up all the time that haven't even been given names yet. If you have an undiagnosed disorder, it's especially important to believe in yourself. If you feel that intuitively something is wrong, it likely is. You can maintain your dignity even if others doubt you.

"Mainstream" Diagnoses

When Louise, age forty-six, started having vision problems, she sought help from her doctor. After ruling out eye problems, he ran some standard tests which indicated that she had diabetes. She was given a special diet and a home-testing devise to keep an eye on her blood sugar.

While Louise's disability is a societally recognized one, she still faced judgment from others. Her mother admonished her for "causing" her diabetes by being overweight. A good friend suggested that the diabetes may have developed now because of a relationship breakup. Several people offered unsolicited advice.

You, like Louise, may have a traditional diagnosis, such as diabetes, asthma, or migraines. While it may take some time to rule out other diseases, eventually your doctor can diagnose the problem. You can locate numerous books and articles on the disorder; there are national organizations with local chapters for assistance and support. Most people will recognize your problem when you reveal it.

Even having an easily understood problem, however, can prove challenging. Others assume that stress caused your symptoms. You're inundated with suggestions about alternative treatments. Feeling ashamed to have ended up with a chronic illness, you may blame yourself for being "weak." But it's important to remember that you didn't cause your problem. Many people are vulnerable to contracting health problems, especially if there's a genetic component.

Progressive or Life-Threatening Illnesses

Jenny, a fifty-two-year-old editor, just returned from her second hospitalization this year. Diagnosed with lupus, her kidneys began to fail. While strong medication had generally kept the disease under control, she's had several frightening health crises. She feels like her body, once a friend, has turned on her.

Having a life-threatening illness—such as lupus, cancer, AIDS, or sickle-cell anemia—is extremely difficult. There may be no way to predict the course of your illness. Yet, not only do you contend with significant physical discomfort and uncertainty, you have to tolerate the sometimes insensitive responses from others. For instance, cancer survivors are routinely described as repressed, weak, and passive—the so-called "cancer personality." On top of having cancer, you're now labeled by some as having a deficient personality. If you have a life-threatening illness, you may also be subject to facile explanations about why you've become ill. If you feel as if others are directly or indirectly blaming you for "causing" your disease, keep in mind that doing this allows them to avoid feeling their anxiety about becoming ill themselves. They may think, consciously or unconsciously, "I won't get cancer because I'm not repressed," or "Lupus sufferers can't handle stress, but I can."

Some problems, like multiple sclerosis (MS), may not be life threatening, but they're instead progressive, meaning symptoms may worsen over time. Yet often the prognosis is unknown. Some seemingly able-bodied people have multiple sclerosis, while others with the disease are confined to wheelchairs. Living with a potentially progressive illness can cause much anxiety and distress, but your suffering may not be easily recognized by others. You may look "normal," which can make it more difficult for some of your friends and family to truly accept that your illness may progress.

If you have a progressive or life-threatening illness, remember that it's understandable if you feel anxious. It helps to learn as much as you can about your disorder to see if you can identify triggers and flare-ups. Connecting with others who share your illness or circumstances may also help.

Uncommon Disorders

Brad was a musician until he awoke one day with a loud ringing in his right ear. After a few days, the piercing noise spread to his left ear, and ordinary sounds hurt. Brad had developed tinnitus (noises in the ear) and hyperacusis (an inability to tolerate normal sounds).

Not only was his ear disorder disabling, but he was frustrated by others' reactions. "Hyper what?" his brother asked, then added, "Becoming a bit of a hypochondriac, bro?" His doctor declared that hyperacusis was extremely rare with no cure. "Change professions and wear ear plugs," he offered. When Brad asked his dentist about whether the drill could exacerbate the problem, his dentist admitted he'd never heard of hyperacusis.

Some disorders, like hyperacusis, are rare. Because they're uncommon, few people have heard of the problem. While it's understandable that friends and family may be ignorant, it's especially distressing when some health care professionals are also in the dark. It can be troubling when you can't find your hidden disability listed in popular health books, making it an uphill climb to locate information about your prognosis and appropriate treatment.

When you're stuck with a rare disorder, you're always explaining it to other people. You wonder whether others believe you. As Brad relates:

> When I told this woman I had hyperacusis and tinnitus, she gave me a blank look. I ended up having to explain for ten minutes what the problem was all about. She, of course, had a lot of questions, many of which I couldn't answer. By the end of the conversation, I got the distinct sense she thought I was off my rocker.

If you have an uncommon disorder, it's important to realize that you're vulnerable to skepticism. You may have to describe your disorder to people so that they'll understand. Even so, people often question disorders they've never heard of before. While you may want to educate some people, your job isn't to single-handedly convince the general public about the existence of your hidden disability. You can choose to share information or not.

Assume responsibility for learning as much as you can. Brad, for instance, found out about an excellent hyperacusis organization started by someone with the problem. He learned about new treatments, such as innovative ear devices. He started writing letters to other hyperacusis sufferers and no longer felt so odd and out of place.

"Socially Unacceptable" Disorders

Bob, a twenty-seven-year-old high school teacher, started noticing changes in his bowel habits. He had diarrhea for no apparent reason, even blood in his stool. Alarmed, he saw a specialist who diagnosed him with inflammatory bowel disease (IBD). While IBD is a recognized disorder, Bob was embarrassed to tell anyone. At work, he endured painful bouts, too ashamed to ask for increased bathroom breaks. Since he didn't want to tell friends about his problem, he isolated himself from others.

While it can feel embarrassing to have almost any hidden disability, some disorders are particularly stigmatizing. Intestinal disorders like IBD can feel shameful to disclose. This is also true for illnesses involving "private parts," such as the rectum, bladder, or reproductive organs. Our culture still maintains a taboo against discussing normal functions, such as elimination and urination. Sharing with another person that you have chronic rectal pain, for instance, leaves you open to teasing, giggles, and callous remarks. It's hard enough to be in pain. But it's especially unfair to be the object of ridicule or aversion.

If you have a "socially unacceptable" disability, try to go easy on yourself. Endometriosis or interstitial cystitis are just as real and debilitating as lower back pain. You have nothing to be embarrassed about. While our culture maintains a juvenile attitude about normal human functions, you don't have to personalize this reaction.

If people make insensitive remarks, realize that this shows their immaturity and discomfort. At the same time, you don't have to allow yourself to be the receptacle of ridicule. Share your problem with sensitive and understanding people. If someone teases you, let him or her know that these comments are hurtful and inappropriate.

Many people are living with socially stigmatizing disorders. You don't always know about it because people are reticent and hide their experiences. It can be empowering and comforting to talk with others who share or understand your illness. Many people join support groups that meet in person or over the Internet. There are often web sites where you can freely communicate and ventilate.

Pain Problems

Rochelle had worked as an executive secretary for ten years without any pain in her wrists. But when her office converted to computers several years ago, her wrists and forearms began aching and tingling. When she began dropping things and had trouble opening bottles, she became alarmed and saw her doctor. He diagnosed her with a repetitive strain injury (RSI). When Rochelle asked for more breaks from word processing, her request received an icy reception from co-workers, who assumed she was trying to slack off from work.

Once uncommon, repetitive strain injuries (RSI) now comprise 60 percent of all work-related illnesses and cost the economy twenty billion dollars a year (Wolkomir 1994). Most sufferers develop RSIs from repetitive movements on the job, such as computer or factory work. The effect on work and home is devastating. Not only are RSIs physically painful and debilitating, but the disorder may prevent you from working in your usual occupation.

If you have an RSI, you might also face skepticism and ridicule from others who accuse you of exaggerating or seeking special treatment. While RSI sufferers are often seen as malingering, ironically it's often the hardest workers who are at risk of developing an RSI. If you're a workaholic who takes few breaks and ignores initial signs of trouble, you may be in line for an RSI. This is not to say that only workaholics get RSIs. Everyone's body is different. One preventative measure you can take, however, is to keep in mind how important it is to listen and respond to early warning signs of pain.

There are numerous other disorders that also cause pain. Some cancer survivors, for instance, undergo medical treatments that eliminate the disease—only to end up with chronic pain that confounds doctors. Many chronic illnesses, such as lupus, rheumatoid arthritis, cancer, and chronic fatigue syndrome, are painful. This type of pain is usually frightening because it may signal a serious flare-up and sometimes even leads to hospitalization. Or you may have injured yourself and consequently ended up with chronic pain. Perhaps you were in an accident and your pain has never remitted. Some people with this experience have recently been diagnosed with myofascial pain syndrome (MPS), another controversial diagnosis that elicits skepticism.

Living with pain wears down your body and spirits. It is depressing to wake up each day and feel familiar uncomfortable sensations. People in your life may misunderstand your pain. They wonder why, a year after your car accident, you still hurt. Friends suggest quick fixes, like medications or the latest bodywork craze. Even doctors may not understand; if your MRI looks normal, you may be perceived as exaggerating. You may be dispatched to a psychotherapist to look for psychological reasons for your pain.

If you suffer from chronic pain, you'll find chapter 10 particularly helpful, as it is devoted to the causes and treatments of pain. Make a commitment to try some of the exercises to reduce pain. And remember: Even if the cause of your pain can't be determined by medical tests, it's still real. Some pain conditions resist treatment and linger, even when the original injury has healed. Don't blame or degrade yourself for still being in pain. While you can't always control the physical pain you experience, you can minimize your emotional suffering.

Psychological Disorders

Mindy, a twenty-nine-year-old artist, had experienced mood swings since adolescence. Her manic highs, where she'd charge thousands of dollars on her credit cards and suddenly leave home for days, cost her two divorces. Mindy's low periods landed her in bed for days, contemplating suicide. Her new boyfriend insisted that she see a psychiatrist, who diagnosed her with bipolar disorder (manic depression). Her moods are now stabilized with medication.

Mood disorders, such as bipolar disorder and depression, are common conditions that strike millions of people. Other psychological disabilities include attention deficit disorder, obsessive compulsive disorder, Tourette's syndrome, and anxiety disorders. For years, experts believed that these problems were the result of trauma or poor parenting. Mothers, especially, were routinely faulted for being either overly attached or too distant. Psychotherapists probed for the early childhood wound that caused the bout of schizophrenia or depression.

While the environment affects human behavior, recent studies reveal a bio-chemical basis for many psychiatric disorders. However, there's still an enormous stigma attached to having one of them. People may view you as morally deficient, unbalanced, and the product of a dysfunctional family. Some people avoid you, fearing your condition will be "contagious" or that you are somehow dangerous. Other people may "psychoanalyze" you, even if they lack any scientific knowledge regarding your disorder. Well-meaning but misguided people may pity you or fear that you'll go "crazy" on them.

Maintaining self-esteem may seem like an impossible task. But it's important that you try. You don't have to accept the stigma attached to a psychiatric disorder. Nor are you obliged to share your condition with the world. Choose who to tell and when. Reach out to others with similar disabilities. And search for effective treatment; some of the newer medications boast fewer side effects than the older varieties.

In this book, we will provide a variety of examples of people living with psychiatric hidden disabilities. While the scope of this book does not include all of the issues specific to psychiatric disabilities, we feel that much of the information is applicable to both psychological and physical issues.

What Causes Hidden Disabilities?

If you ask ten people why you're ill, you could potentially get as many as ten different opinions. Your acupuncturist may blame your kidney meridian. Your chiropractor says you're out of alignment. Your medical doctor suspects your problems are psychosomatic. And your therapist thinks your feelings regarding your parents' divorce when you were ten are the cause of your problems, disregarding the possibility of a physiological component or cause.

Whom to believe? You desperately want to know why you're sick or in pain. Yet it's perplexing when everyone has a different hunch. Some theories seem far-fetched, such as "you're being punished for an infraction in a past life." Many of the explanations feel overwhelming, like when your therapist says you have a "dependent personality" and internalize your suffering. How do you change your dependent personality if you've lived with it for twenty or even fifty years? These theories take a toll on your morale. You might start wondering if there's anything about you that's not broken.

In this section, we'll describe some of the common theories about what causes hidden disabilities. You've probably heard many of them before. Some beliefs make you feel reassured; others contribute to self-blame. We'll also discuss how to cope when you feel disheartened by these theories.

Medical Model

Vanessa, a twenty-five-year-old aspiring actress, developed nerve pain down her arm after a car accident. Her primary care physician ran tests but they came up negative. He referred her to a neurologist who said her pain was psychological due to the trauma of the crash. He prescribed pain medications, but these upset her stomach. Several months later, Vanessa's foot was aching. Her doctor referred her to a podiatrist. He performed X rays, said her foot was fine, and sent her to a physical therapist.

When Vanessa developed migraines, she again returned to her regular doctor. She asked if there could be a connection among all of her symptoms. He answered no, that there was no known syndrome that involved arm and foot pain plus migraines. Puzzled and wary, he suggested she see a psychotherapist.

Vanessa's experience illustrates many of the features of the medical model. Symptoms are diagnosed by medical tests and physical examinations. If the symptoms meet the criteria for a disorder, a diagnosis is made. Medication is prescribed to eliminate the pain, even though it may cause unwanted side effects. Various symptoms are often seen as separate. Specialists view the problem only from their area of expertise. If no diagnosis can be made, many doctors suspect that the problem is psychologically based.

The medical model is pretty straightforward. You injure yourself, and therefore your body hurts. A particular organ breaks down, so you contract a disease. You have faulty genes or are otherwise susceptible to illness. Surgery and drugs are used to battle the "enemy"—your illness or pain. If a problem isn't alleviated in a set amount of time, doctors may question whether your emotions are interfering with recovery.

This model is sometimes sufficient to help manage or alleviate the problem. Disorders like diabetes can be determined through tests. Treatment is standard and consists of a change of diet, exercise, and medications. Doctors can predict which organs may be damaged by the diabetes, and there are various treatments to try.

But what about when the hidden disability is unusual and puzzling? Vanessa's symptoms, for instance, did not fit the profile of a particular disorder. She was sent from one specialist to another without anyone trying to link the problems together. When no one could figure out why she was in pain, her problems were labeled psychological.

When a hidden disability is not easily diagnosed, you can end up feeling lost and misunderstood. Your days become consumed with visiting new specialists and enduring medical tests. You experiment with different kinds of pills, some of which cause new symptoms. When no one can find the answer, you may wonder if you're losing your mind. Yet, intuitively, you know that something is really wrong, that you aren't imagining your symptoms.

If you're in this situation, remember: Don't consider doctors to be all-knowing. They generally know a great deal about many disorders and very little about others. Medical science is still in its infancy regarding chronic pain and immunological disorders. While it's worth trying some treatments, be wary. Don't volunteer for risky tests and medications without much forethought and consideration. Research all your options, check out information on the Internet, and purchase some good health books. In chapter 11, we offer further guidance in working well with health care professionals.

Psychosomatic Model

If you have a hidden disability, you're undoubtedly familiar with this theory. It goes like this: Your physical symptoms are really psychological. You're simply expressing unresolved emotional issues through your body, which is called "somaticizing." Since it's hard to express your internal pain, your body exhibits it through symptoms. For instance, you have chronic pain because you're unassertive. Or your fatigue and flu-like symptoms mean you're sick of your life. When you finally work through your psychological problems, your pain will vanish.

Vanessa's psychotherapist advocated this theory. He told Vanessa that her nerve pain meant that she was "nervous" about becoming an actress. Her pain provided a convenient excuse to avoid pursuing her dream. He believed that she derived much attention from her "performance" of being a pain victim. After months of exploring her nervousness and self-doubt, Vanessa felt more confident about pursuing acting. The problem was that her chronic pain hadn't decreased a bit.

A popular proponent of this theory is John Sarno, a medical doctor, who asserts that most chronic pain in the body springs from repressed anxiety and anger. He says that fibromyalgia, for instance, is all psychosomatic (Sarno 1991). His treatment is simple: Ignore the pain, return to all your old activities, and figure out why you're anxious and angry. Sarno declares that the vast majority of patients who follow his plan become symptom-free, although he concedes that his statistics only include patients who embrace his thinking.

Sarno suggests a simple test to determine whether your symptoms are psychosomatic—take a vacation. Go hiking or biking like you've longed to since your disability began troubling you. Relax, swim, rent a canoe, ski. Ignore any pain sensations. After the trip is over, see how you feel. Sarno cites numerous examples of people who are "cured" of their pain after their trip. While Sarno doesn't emphasize the hazards of trying this, be forewarned that you're taking a big risk. Many patients with hidden disabilities who overdid exercise have ended up flat on their backs.

Another champion of this theory is Carla Cantor, who believes that virtually all pain is psychosomatic. In her book, she dubs chronic fatigue and fibromyalgia sufferers as hypochondriacs (Cantor 1996). Using her own experience as a victim of chronic pain who was "cured" by Prozac, Cantor believes that people suffering from stomach ailments and immune problems are also manifesting emotional problems.

Cantor cites as proof the fact that many pain patients gain relief from antidepressants. However, she neglects to mention that chronic pain, like depression, reduces levels of a brain chemical called serotonin, which produces feelings of well-being. Thus, Prozac can help sufferers of chronic pain because it increases serotonin. Also, antidepressants for pain are generally prescribed at a much lower dose than for people suffering from clinical depression. Many people with fibromyalgia, for instance, take Elavil, an antidepressant frequently prescribed for pain reduction. Dosages are commonly about 10 mg. The therapeutic dose for depression is 150 to 300 mg.

If you suffer from a hidden disability, chances are that some people in your life consider your symptoms psychosomatic. Maintaining your self-confidence, not to mention your temper, when interacting with these people can pose a challenge. It doesn't help when you read articles and books by authors who only reinforce your worst fear that you're a hypochondriac.

While there are certainly people who somaticize their symptoms, the vast majority of those with chronic pain, illness, or psychological problems have real illnesses. Robert Taylor, a medical doctor, argues persuasively against assuming that vague physical problems are psychosomatic (Taylor 1982). He devotes an entire book to what he calls "medical masquerades," that is, disorders that are viewed as psychological when the patient actually has a physical problem. He cites studies where 10 percent to 46 percent of psychiatric patients actually had undiagnosed physical problems. Once treated, their psychological problems were alleviated. Taylor states, "The casual use of the concept of somatization or the term *hysterical* is to be avoided; such practice opens the door to tragic mistakes in critical assessment."

He cautions clinicians to be very careful before attaching a psychosomatic label to a patient. In fact, he believes that one of these criteria should be met before seriously considering the diagnosis of somatization:

1. The complaint arises out of a stressful situation, such as an unhappy relationship or work stress. Once the stressor is identified and dealt with, the medical problem disappears. Even if the stressor persists, the symptoms generally dissipate on their own.

2. There's a sudden loss of a specific body function, for instance, the right arm becoming paralyzed or abrupt blindness. There aren't widespread bodily complaints. The onset is often dramatic. Generally, function is restored after a period of time.

3. The problem provides an answer to a severe life problem. A dramatic example would be poet Maya Angelou's becoming mute as a teenager after a relative murdered the man who raped her (Angelou 1997). She was horrified about the tragic consequences of disclosing the rape. Speaking felt dangerous. Once Angelou was able to heal from this trauma, she regained her ability to speak.

If you don't meet Taylor's criteria, chances are that you are not a hypochondriac. While your symptoms may seem vague and puzzling, they are real. While others may trivialize your problem, it's most important that you believe in yourself. While you can't control how others perceive you, you can believe in yourself.

Secondary Gain

This theory is a close relative to the psychosomatic one. It holds that you're not healing for a reason; you're benefiting in some way from being ill. When you're no longer gaining financial or emotional rewards from having a hidden disability, you'll get well. Vanessa's therapist was an advocate of this theory. He thought her pain symptoms were a psychosomatic response that allowed her to avoid facing her fear of acting.

Most therapists are well-versed in this popular theory. They may ask you what you're gaining from being ill. But mental health professionals are not the only ones who may subscribe to this way of thinking. Janice Wittenberg, an MCS and CFIDS sufferer, devotes several pages in her otherwise helpful book to how people often benefit from being ill (Wittenberg 1996). She suggests that illness may make you feel more interesting and special; you're also offered a convenient escape from responsibilities.

While there are likely a small number of people who derive benefits from having a hidden disability, most people would like nothing better than to get well. Your illness is more likely to make you feel alienated and weak than special. You're probably distressed by being dependent, and you'd likely relish feeling in control of your life again. The small amount of money you may receive from public assistance or from family is no consolation for living with pain or illness. When your illness flares up, you feel despondent. Good days bring hopefulness and relief.

It's unfair when others accuse you of causing your plight or having the power to "overcome" your disability. Being disabled is difficult enough without having people assume that you could get better if you wanted to enough. If there are people in your life who espouse these sentiments and you find that their comments dishearten you, set limits. Try to associate with people who understand that being sick and in pain is burdensome and that your goal is to alleviate and cope with your disability, not prolong it.

Alternative or New Age Theories

Many of Vanessa's friends held so-called New Age beliefs. Here are a few she's heard:

- "You have pain because there's a lesson you need to learn. Once you learn this lesson, you'll recover."

- "You've been holding in all of your emotions, and that's why you're ill."

- "Your life is out of balance. Doing some deep spiritual work will cure your illness."

- "When you're ready and willing to heal, you will."

- "Your illness is a wonderful gift."

- "You're sick because of bad karma."

While Vanessa's friends were well-meaning, their comments left her feeling blamed, inadequate, and guilty. She felt inferior, as if she'd ended up ill because she mishandled her emotions. She worried about whether she'd ever learn the "lesson" and get well. She resented her friends insisting that her pain was a gift when it felt like a misfortune. Vanessa felt overwhelmed at the monumental task of becoming "more spiritual," but was afraid that if she didn't do this the way her friends were suggesting, she'd never get any better.

When Vanessa joined a pain support group, she learned that illness can happen to anyone. Given that there were group members from every walk of life, she understood that pain was a part of life. She realized that there were no simple answers to why her pain developed or persisted. Vanessa stopped listening to her friends' theories, which she found disheartening, and started trusting her own intuition.

There are numerous writers who promote the New Age way of thinking. Carolyn Myss, a popular speaker, writer, and "medical intuitive," believes that there's a deeper meaning for almost any disorder (Myss and Sheahy 1993). According to her, developing multiple sclerosis means you're storing resentment and have dependency issues. Epileptics experience seizures because of explosive rage. Rheumatoid arthritis patients are passive and angry. Those with lupus hate themselves and feel controlled. Given the enormous numbers of people with dependency issues, rage, and passivity, Myss neglects to explain why only some people get these disorders. Her theories also fail to illuminate why many dependent or angry people don't develop hidden disabilities.

Bernie Siegel, a best-selling author, makes this pronouncement: "The simple truth is, happy people generally don't get sick" (Siegel 1986). According to Siegel, by becoming a more fulfilled and spiritually aware person, illness may spontaneously vanish. Siegel never makes it clear how joyful babies and toddlers contract illnesses and even die young.

Illness and other misfortunes can occur to anyone at any time; this is part of the human experience. Tragedy strikes good families as well as corrupt ones. Lou Gehrig, the sports hero, succumbed to amyotrophic lateral sclerosis (ALS) in his thirties. Linda McCartney, the partner to Beatles' member Paul McCartney, was a loving mother and a committed humanitarian, yet she died in her fifties from breast cancer. Innocent children develop AIDS and numerous other illnesses.

Is it really fair and compassionate to assume that these people were somehow "chosen" for a particular teaching? Or that their lives weren't spiritual enough? Or that they weren't happy? Rabbi Harold Kushner reminds us that sometimes "bad things happen to good people" even though there are no logical reasons why (Kushner 1990). He was motivated to write after his teenage son died from a painful and debilitating disease.

Happy people can develop hidden disabilities. Unhappy people, even vicious criminals, can enjoy good health until age ninety. In fact, a number of dictators, including Joseph Stalin and Pol Pot, lived until old age. Attaching blame to those who become ill is misguided, naive, and hurtful.

You may be inundated with well-meaning people who are imploring you to become more spiritual, figure out why you became sick in the first place, and learn to heal yourself. Their comments may depress and discourage you. Don't let them. It's important that you don't give away your power. Remember that there are no simple answers to why you've developed a hidden disability. Given that you've expended much energy to becoming well, there may be no quick fixes. Illness is not a punishment or a disgrace. It doesn't set you apart from other people. Crises, problems, and pain are all part of being alive.

Lifestyle Theory

In a nutshell, this theory contends that you are what you eat. So if you've spent the last few decades consuming copious amounts of fatty foods, drinking too much alcohol, and exercising rarely, your lifestyle has made you sick. Recreational drug use, stress, overwork, and cigarettes supposedly increase your chances of developing a hidden disability.

This theory is compelling in some ways. The overweight person does have a higher risk of diabetes, heart disease, and back pain. Being out of shape can make it easier to pull muscles and slower to recover. Smoking causes emphysema and cancer. Yet there are plenty of healthy senior citizens who've lived unhealthy lifestyles. And many health-conscious people end up with a hidden disability.

Why one person becomes ill and another doesn't is a complex matter. Lifestyle may be a factor for some people. For others, genetics and the environment play bigger roles. Each person is unique. One person may be very sensitive to stress and succumb to illness. Another can work sixty hours a week, smoke cigarettes, and infrequently exercise, yet live to a robust old age.

It's helpful to evaluate your lifestyle, but do so without self-blame. If you think that being overweight has contributed to your knee pain, commit yourself to losing weight. But realize that there are numerous reasons why you're overweight in the first place. Many scientists now believe that you have a genetic "blueprint" that predisposes you to become a certain weight. Also, personality traits and difficult life experiences can make you eat compulsively to comfort yourself. Try to be compassionate with yourself as you seek a healthier lifestyle.

Environmental Theory

Consider these facts:

- Rachel Carson sounded the alarm about the dangers of pesticides in her seminal book, *Silent Spring,* written in 1962. Yet, all of these years later, there are four times as many pesticides now in use—over fifty thousand (Steinman 1990). Rachel Carson died of bone cancer in 1964.

- Only 10 percent of all pesticides have been tested for potential health effects (Elkington et al. 1990).

- Children living in houses where pesticides are used inside and out are nine times as likely to develop leukemia as those in pesticide-free houses (Lawson 1993).

- Twenty thousand Americans each year develop cancer due to pesticides (Lawson 1993).

- At the turn of the century, cancer accounted for less than 1 percent of all deaths. Today that figure is 20 percent (Steinman 1990).

Reading these figures, it's hard to ignore the enormous hazards of chemicals. Not only are pesticides suspect, but also there's continual exposure to risky toxins at home, work, and play. Almost everything—including food, water, furniture, carpeting, soaps, shampoos, bedding, and electronic devices—contains chemicals.

The health problems associated with chemicals don't happen overnight. Each exposure is stored in the blood and body fat, and the chemicals accumulate. Though everyone is exposed to countless chemicals and pollutants from birth, some people eventually experience "chemical overload." This is when the body breaks down and can no longer tolerate even small exposures. The numbers of people with heightened sensitivity to toxins aren't small. Conservative estimates are 15 percent of the U.S. population, or 37 million Americans. Some studies have produced figures as high as 66 percent (Radetsky 1997).

Toxins cause not only multiple chemical sensitivities. Alzheimer's disease, a degenerative brain disease, has risen rapidly and may be linked to aluminum and mercury exposure (Steinman 1990). The rates of asthma and allergies, especially among young children, have skyrocketed. Autoimmune disorders are on the rise, as are neurological diseases like ALS, popularly known as Lou Gehrig's disease.

It's likely, then, that many hidden disabilities result from the poisoning of the earth. The chronically ill may be "canaries in the mine." Miners would bring canaries into mines, and when the canaries stopped singing or died, the miners knew it was time to flee. These types of hidden disabilities can be ridiculed or shunned, or the predicament can be seen as a warning and a reason to reduce the number of chemicals in use. People with multiple chemical sensitivities and similar disabilities may be the modern-day version of the proverbial canary.

Integrative Model

We believe in a subtle interplay of the mind, the body, and the environment, in addition to any number of unknown or seemingly unrelated factors (e.g., accidents, lifestyle, stress, genes) precipitating illness and injury. We call this the "integrative model." When using this model, it's important to remember that each person is unique. One person may go through a terrible trauma, compromising his or her immune functioning and becoming ill. Yet another person may also suffer through the same exact kind of trauma and still thrive. Viktor Frankl, for example, survived the horrors of Nazi Germany, was imprisoned in Auschwitz and Dachau, and lost his wife and most of his family. Yet, prior to his death in 1997 at age ninety-two, he was a prolific writer and founder of an influential school of psychology called logotherapy.

Myths about Hidden Disabilities

Myth: Stress causes hidden disabilities.

Reality: There's some evidence that stress and trauma increase susceptibility to illness or injury. However, why one person develops a disability is complicated.

Myth: If my doctor can't figure out what's wrong with me, then my problem must be all in my head.

Reality: Many hidden disabilities are never diagnosed. Yet if you believe intuitively that something is wrong, it probably is.

Myth: If a person remains sick, he or she must be benefiting in some way.

Reality: Having a hidden disability is crushing to the mind and spirit. There are many more losses than benefits.

Myth: Hidden disabilities strike those who are depressed or weak.

Reality: A hidden disability can affect anyone at any time.

Myth: Developing a disability is a wonderful gift.

Reality: Disabilities are difficult and painful. Whether a person views it as a gift or not is highly individual.

Myth: If you develop a hidden disability, your life is over.

Reality: You can still live a full life even if you have a hidden disability.

Does this mean that the person who becomes ill is inferior or deficient? Not at all. It simply implies that some people are more susceptible than others to developing a hidden disability. There are many forces at play in any human life. Why one person remains healthy while another becomes ill is often a mystery.

While human beings try to control everything through knowledge, there are many aspects of life that no one can fully understand. Scientists trap and tag birds to understand flight patterns; yet, humans can never know the mystery of why birds fly. There are innumerable other such enigmas such as: What's the purpose of life? Why are we here? These are universal, essential questions of living. Why one person's life is plagued with difficulty while another appears charmed is a puzzle that no one can answer with absolute certainty. While people in your life swear that it's your diet or your emotions, the truth is that in many cases, no one really knows.

You may not be able to solve this mystery. Nevertheless, you can learn from it. Even if you endure daily pain, you can still live a full life. You're not responsible for your illness, but you are responsible for your life. You can become embittered and self-hating, or you can learn to live well even if you have a hidden disability. It's up to you to take the challenge.

This book offers you ideas and tips on how to cope. By grieving your losses, adapting to change, and counteracting negative habits, you can accept your life. By recognizing your inner strength, you can love yourself in spite of having a hidden disability. And in the end, perhaps that is the true meaning of "healing": having courage under fire, learning to love yourself, and making the best of whatever life throws your way.

Reminders

You are not alone; millions of others are living with hidden disabilities.

People may offer various theories about why you're ill or in pain, but no one knows for sure why you've developed a hidden disability.

You are not responsible for causing your hidden disability, but you are responsible for how you live your life now.

You can still enjoy your life even if you're saddled with chronic pain, illness, or a psychiatric disability.

CHAPTER 2

The Stages of Grief: Working toward Acceptance

When it finally hit me that I had fibromyalgia—that it was something chronic with no instant cure—I sank into such a dark hole. I felt like a part of me had died.

—Jane, age twenty-eight

When you hear the word "grief," you probably tend to think of death. Yet to live with a hidden disability is to suffer a profound sense of loss. Like Jane, it can be experienced as a kind of death. And in some ways it is. When you're healthy, your life generally feels unlimited and boundless. When you're forced to curtail or modify activities, you grieve. This isn't to say that there aren't precious lessons and gifts from having a hidden disability. But loss is an inherent part of illness and pain.

There's also a more subtle type of loss—the loss of belief in your own infallibility, that you can stay healthy and vigorous forever. By developing a hidden disability, you're confronted with some hard lessons: No one lives forever, and you cannot always control your destiny. This truth can offer you much wisdom about living in the present and appreciating moments of diminished pain.

Elisabeth Kubler-Ross was one of the first professionals to write about grief, and her stages of grief are quoted widely. While she wrote them to describe the process of dying, they apply as well to a hidden disability. She says that you go through different stages when you experience loss. These stages are: denial and isolation, anger, bargaining, depression, and acceptance (Kubler-Ross 1997).

However, with a hidden disability, the stages of grief look different than when facing death. One reason is that the stages keep repeating themselves as you move through relapses, healthy periods, and new symptoms. You may think you've truly accepted your disability and then, during a flare-up, you become depressed and disheartened. It may be hard to accept your disability fully if other people in your life don't validate or acknowledge your condition.

Here's a description of the stages of grief as they apply to having a hidden disability. While mourning is a normal process, it's important not to get stuck in any one stage. Getting entrenched in anger or depression is unhealthy for your spirit as well as your body. If you find that you are getting stuck, remember to reach out for support from those you trust.

Stage One: Denial and Isolation

Denial

Catherine stops taking her medication for bipolar (manic-depressive) disorder because she's feeling better. Daniel, who has multiple sclerosis, walks much farther than usual and falls on his face, sustaining deep cuts and bruises. Jackie goes skiing even after being diagnosed with a herniated disc and is bedridden upon return.

These people are in denial of their disability: Catherine believes she's cured, Daniel wants to forget that he has physical limitations, and Jackie refuses to give up her beloved sport. Denial is what's called a "defense mechanism," which your mind uses to guard against a frightening and threatening experience. Through denial, you try to allay anxiety.

Denial is normal with any new diagnosis. You run from one doctor to another to find a quick cure or a more benign diagnosis. You continue your relentless work pace, refusing to slow down. In fact, denial can be a useful defense at first, allowing the reality of a hidden disability to slowly penetrate, reducing the chances of feeling overwhelmed. However, if denial continues for very long, problems like those Catherine, Daniel, and Jackie experienced may occur. Part of self-care when you have a hidden disability involves tuning in carefully to what your body needs. Ignoring early warning signs and pretending a disability doesn't really exist can lead to more flare-ups and a longer recovery time.

Denial can be both healthy and unhealthy. Healthy denial allows you to continue to live life without obsessing about your hidden disability. For instance, if John, who is HIV positive, ruminates all day about the future, he'll be unable to enjoy what he can do now. Yet denial can also lead to more problems if unnecessary risks are taken.

To discover the role of denial in your life, take this quiz. Just circle the number under the correct answer:

1. I acknowledge to myself that I have a hidden disability.

Always	*Sometimes*	*Never*
0	1	2

2. I acknowledge to others that I have a hidden disability.

Always	*Sometimes*	*Never*
0	1	2

3. I tend to overdo my activities.

Always	*Sometimes*	*Never*
0	1	2

4. I have had flare-ups caused by overdoing it.

Always	*Sometimes*	*Never*
0	1	2

Now count up your scores by adding up the numbers underneath the answer you circled.

0–3: You rarely engage in denial.

4–6: You occasionally engage in denial and are at some risk of overdoing your activities.

6–8: You engage in denial quite a bit and are frequently overdoing activities.

You should make an effort to understand the role of denial in your hidden disability. Consider whether denial is helping or hurting you. If, for instance, you have frequent flare-ups because you overdo things, then you need to acknowledge that your body requires special attention. On the other hand, if you engage in denial to not dwell on the scary aspects of your illness, denial may be helping.

If, after taking a look at your denial, you feel you're engaging in it in an unhealthy way, there are a number of steps you can take. First, understand why your denial persists. Start by completing these statements:

1. If I admitted to myself that I have a hidden disability, I would feel _____

_____

2. If I admitted to myself that I have a hidden disability, others in my life would feel _____

and react this way: _____

_____

3. These people in my life are denying my hidden disability: _____

_____

Their denial makes me feel _____

_____

_____

4. The hardest part about acknowledging that I have a hidden disability is

_____

_____

5. It would be helpful for me to acknowledge having a hidden disability because

_____

_____

Once you take a look at what's behind your continued denial, you can break through it. For example, Steven, a thirty-year-old architect, continued to deny that he had ulcerative colitis, even going on a trip to Mexico during a flare-up, which plunged him into such an inflammatory state that he required hospitalization for ten days and high dosages of steroids. By asking himself these questions, he realized that acknowledging his disability meant feeling powerless. Steven has always tried to control his life, from his marriage to his kids to his job. While being diagnosed with colitis was devastating, he learned a valuable lesson: He can't control everything. And by being a control freak, he was damaging relationships with loved ones, as well as his own health.

Once you understand what purpose denial is serving, you can talk to yourself realistically. For instance, Steven can say to himself, "I have a hidden disability that needs special care. But I'm still the same person I've always been. I need to control what I can and let go of the rest." By acknowledging the disability, coupled with calming and comforting phrases, you, like Steven, can offset denial.

When Rose, a thirty-four-year-old mother of two with an undiagnosed immune problem, asked herself these questions, she realized that she was denying her symptoms because her husband refused to accept her hidden disability. He believed that her immune problems were due to stress and admonished her to take better care of herself. Being an unassertive person, Rose minimized her symptoms rather than face a confrontation with her husband.

Isolation

Along with denial, isolation is also considered part of the first stage in the grieving process. It's natural to withdraw during times of great distress. If you've recently been diagnosed and you feel less sociable, remember that this is one of the many "normal" responses. But when does isolation turn to loneliness? And can loneliness impede healing?

The benefits of companionship and social support have been well-documented. In a landmark 1989 study of women with advanced breast cancer, David Spiegel found that women who attended cancer support groups lived twice as long as those who didn't. Other research has shown that even having a pet aids the health and longevity of the elderly.

It's important, then, to notice whether you are isolating yourself. One way to evaluate your social support is to ask yourself these questions.

1. Do you have at least one good friend whom you can turn to? _____

2. How many good friends did you have before you developed your hidden disability? _____ How many do you have now? _____

3. How satisfied are you with the quality of your relationships? _____

   _____

4. Has this changed since developing your hidden disability? _____

5. If you have few friendships, or if you find the ones you have unsatisfying, what do you attribute this to? _____

   _____

6. What are some things that you might be doing to hurt your relationships with others? _____

   _____

7. What are some steps that you can take to improve your current relationships?

   _____

   _____

8. What are some steps that you can take to reach out to more people and make new friends? _____

   _____

The answers to these questions may help you to better understand your relationships, especially if they've changed since you've developed a hidden disability. Perhaps friends and family are more distant. They may feel uncomfortable around you, not knowing what to say or do. People might also withdraw because they aren't getting their needs met since the attention is on you.

Notice also what you might be doing to distance yourself from others—perhaps without realizing it. Take the example of Stephanie, who was recently diagnosed with diabetes. When she answered the above questions, she was distressed to see that her social network decreased from ten good friends to two. She blamed her friends for abandoning her and felt embittered. But by honestly answering these questions, she was forced to take a closer look at her own responsibility in alienating her friends.

After Stephanie was diagnosed, she felt not only depressed and angry, but also ashamed to have a disease that required insulin and a special diet. She would rebuff her friends' attempts to cheer her up or to spend time with her without explaining why. After a while, many of her friends, feeling snubbed, stopped calling. By seeing her role in losing friendships, Stephanie could try to restore them. She called one of her closest friends, told her that she missed her, and asked whether they could get together. Stephanie was relieved when her friend said "yes." Stephanie also decided to put effort into meeting new friends. She joined a diabetes support group run by her local hospital. Not only did she cultivate new relationships with others who understood her feelings, but she also began to overcome her feelings of embarrassment.

Stage Two: Anger

> When I started becoming disabled by migraines, I was angry at everyone—at the doctors who kept telling me to just relax, at my friends who would say, "Oh, I get headaches, too," with no sympathy about the agony I was going through. I was mad at God for ruining my life. And I was pissed off at myself for being somehow "defective."
>
> —Michael, age twenty-five

When you lose important pieces of your life, it's natural to become angry. You feel angry at the unfairness of having a hidden disability when others seem to be feeling fine. You resent having to restrict your activities and be careful about everything you do. There are innumerable triggers: people who question your hidden disability, your body not working the way it should, or your money going to doctors rather than vacations.

In addition, you may find that little irritants enrage you. When you were feeling well and someone displaced you in line, you were probably annoyed. Now, with all of the frustration you're dealing with, you're more likely to lose your cool. Your "fuse," meaning your ability to cope with life's frustrations, has probably become significantly shorter. This shortened fuse results from an accumulation of small frustrations while you experience minimal satisfaction and pleasure. Annoyances build up and your fuse ignites.

While understandable, feeling angry much of the time can elevate your blood pressure, tense your muscles, and exacerbate your symptoms. You'll also have more conflicts with loved ones as well as strangers on the street. Consequently, you'll be even more frustrated. Here are some ways to get a handle on your anger.

Anger Self-Test

It helps to assess your anger quotient. Ask yourself the following questions:

1. Am I more irritable than before I developed a hidden disability?
   ____ Yes ____ No

2. Are my loved ones "walking on eggshells" in my presence?
   ____ Yes ____ No

3. Have people remarked that I seem angrier or more frustrated than usual?   ____ Yes ____ No

4. Do I feel angry not just at specific people and situations, but at the world?   ____ Yes ____ No

5. Have I been experiencing increased heartbeat, tense muscles, rapid breathing (unrelated to my hidden disability)?   ____ Yes ____ No

6. Am I smiling and laughing infrequently, yet angry a lot?
   ____ Yes _____ No

7. Do I have a hard time letting go of incidents that anger or frustrate me?
   ____ Yes ____ No

8. Am I using alcohol, drugs, or food to calm me down?
   ____ Yes ____ No

9. Am I angry about something every day?   ____ Yes ____ No

If you answered yes to one or more questions, you feel a heightened degree of anger. While anger is a normal emotion that everyone feels occasionally, it's a problem when you're angry much of the time. Chronic anger can destroy relationships, cause problems at work, and even worsen your symptoms and cause new ones.

Anger versus Hostility

If chronic anger festers and grows, it turns into bitterness and hostility. While anger is an emotion that comes and goes, hostility is a state of ill will against the world. When you're hostile, you see the world as your enemy. You're not just angry at your demanding boss but at all people in authority. You not only silently curse the police officer who ticketed you for speeding, you rant that "all cops are pigs."

For instance, Matthew, a fifty-three-year-old electrician, started out merely angry about having Meniere's disease, a debilitating inner ear condition. He decided he was going to "beat this thing" and used his anger productively to be assertive with doctors, search the Internet for information, and advocate for himself with his health insurance provider.

Yet when all of his hard work didn't stop the vertigo, and he had to take a medical leave from his job, Matthew's anger turned into hostility. He railed against the "stupid doctors who don't know anything" and was rude and impatient to salespeople. His wife tried in vain to point out that his hostility wasn't helping his recovery, not to mention their marriage, but he only exploded in rage. It took her packing up and leaving before Matthew realized his hostility was out of control and that he needed counseling.

Not only can hostility destroy relationships, it can also cause serious health problems such as high blood pressure. Researcher Aron Siegman asked participants to speak about frustrating situations in loud and angry tones or slow and soft ones (Siegman 1996). The blood pressure of those who spoke loudly were in the danger zones, while the slow speakers' were normal. The good news is that when Siegman had the angry speakers change their tone to slow and soft, their blood levels dropped dramatically. He concluded that heart rates drop when you soften your tone.

"Sideways Anger": Passive-Aggressiveness

Loud expressions of anger are not the only unproductive kind. Being passive-aggressive is also destructive to you and to others. Being passive-aggressive means venting anger in a covert, underhanded way. Examples are: refusing sex because you're angry at your partner for spending too much money, muttering underneath your breath within earshot of the person with whom you're angry, "forgetting" to tell someone you'll be late.

In each scenario, the people are angry but aren't being up front about their feelings. Their actions make other people feel confused, distressed, perhaps even angry. Since the anger is masked, the other person usually feels at a loss as to how to respond. Communication breaks down, and conflicts deepen.

Passive-aggressiveness is a harmful and ineffectual way to get your point across. Since your anger remains buried inside, you're still seething. And your relationships with others will undoubtedly suffer. If you tend to be passive-aggressive, figure out when you're angry and let the other person know in a clear and respectful manner.

How to Manage Your Anger

Here are some techniques to control your anger:

The Suit of Armor

Sometimes your fury stems from feeling vulnerable about having a hidden disability. You snap at others in anticipation of rejection or criticism. It helps to create a mental image of wearing a suit of armor that no one can penetrate. You might prefer the image of being in a bubble, or wearing an astronaut suit, or having a white, protective light surrounding you. Say to yourself, "No one can hurt me. I'm protected and safe."

Time-out

No one successfully resolves an issue in the heat of anger. Remove yourself from the situation for a few minutes or even longer. If, for instance, you're furious at your partner for minimizing your symptoms, take a time-out by going for a walk, turning on the TV, calling a friend, or taking a shower. Then, when you've calmed down, you both can discuss your feelings and thoughts.

Talk about It

Raging is not the only way you can hurt your body; suppressing emotions has also been linked to physical problems. However, venting your anger on unfortunate others won't help. In the 1960s, therapists ran encounter groups where members screamed and hit each other with foam bats. Yet researchers later found out that aggression actually makes anger escalate. Wait until you've calmed down. Then talk to the other person about your feelings.

Choose Your Battles

Is it really worth the surge in blood pressure to argue with the salesperson over a one dollar price difference? Do you need to complain yet again about your co-worker's laziness? Will ranting at the slow driver ahead of you add quality to your life? These battles may not be worth your time. By only focusing your energy on a few things, you can help prevent yourself from feeling worn down by constant confrontation.

Productive versus Unproductive Anger

You're irate that your health plan rejected your request to see a specialist. You harness your fury by contacting the state and submitting a formal complaint letter. You also join a local organization devoted to health care reform. Rather than stew or rage, you've successfully redirected your anger toward positive change.

When you use your anger productively, you can feel empowered. In contrast, unproductive anger makes you and others miserable. If, rather than writing the complaint letter, you scream at your teenager that he's a "lazy, selfish SOB" for messing up the bathroom, you'll alienate him and feel guilty. Name-calling, cursing, intimidating, hitting, or degrading others are destructive ways to express anger. Punishing others passive-aggressively by giving them the cold shoulder for days is equally unproductive.

Unproductive anger feels good—at first. You quickly and forcefully release your pent-up emotion and make the other person feel unhappy as well. But before too long, you'll likely feel ashamed, remorseful, and guilty—and find yourself on the receiving end of the other person's anger. It's better to figure out how you are feeling and channel your anger constructively.

See Anger as Information

Does your anger have anything to teach you? Perhaps you're angry at your best friend for pushing you to try a certain treatment. By noticing that you're angry, you realize that you've been passive in setting limits with him. Rather than storing up resentment, you can talk with him and clear the air.

The Most Destructive Type of Anger

Arguably, the most painful and unproductive anger of all is anger toward yourself. You flagellate yourself for ending up with a hidden disability in the first place. You berate yourself for being so "weak" that you have a problem that few acknowledge or understand. You rage at yourself when you have a flare-up. You accuse yourself of not being brave enough if you become depressed.

You may blame yourself because you feel helpless. When you have no one else to be angry with, it's easy to dump on yourself. Self-blame is a means of reestablishing a sense of control. For example, Mark, who suffers from "Gulf War syndrome," believes the experts who say his neurological problems are related to stress. He's angry at himself for succumbing to the syndrome when his buddies didn't. He curses at himself for enlisting in the army in the first place. While his self-anger is demoralizing, the alternative is feeling out of control about having an illness that has stumped all of his specialists.

If your hidden disability resulted from your own actions, your self-anger may be particularly caustic. If you smoked and developed emphysema or had unsafe sex and are now HIV positive, you might spend many unproductive hours chastising yourself. In the final analysis, self-blame changes nothing and depletes you of vital energy. And, if you allow your self-anger to escalate, it will turn into self-hate.

Living with a hidden disability is hard enough without chiding yourself. The antidote is to develop a compassionate attitude toward yourself. You must tame the harsh voice inside you that has been programmed to attack. Recognizing that you are only human, and that humans make mistakes, can help you become kinder toward yourself.

Following are several techniques that can be used to stop self-anger.

"Tape Recorder" Imagery

Imagine that there's a tape recorder in your head with two tapes running. One is your self-anger, which continuously knocks you down. The other is your kind and caring voice, your supporter. Each time you get angry at yourself, envision turning the volume down on the berater and raising the volume on your supporter.

Thought-Stopping

When you start attacking yourself, yell "stop" to yourself. You can also imagine a stop sign or a red light. Don't allow the angry voice to even finish the sentence. When you hear the supporter, you can imagine a green light.

Gaining Perspective

Accept that ups and downs are part of most hidden disabilities. Sometimes you can control flare-ups, and sometimes you can't. Living with a hidden disability is not an exact science.

Self-Compassion

Learn to be compassionate toward yourself. Recognize how much suffering you've experienced—and try not to contribute more. Give yourself credit for how hard you've tried and how much you've done.

A Supportive Voice

Recall somebody in your past or present life who has been supportive. When you start to blame yourself, remember this person's voice and what he or she would say to you.

Stage Three: Bargaining

I'm not a religious person, but after my doctor told me that I had developed severe asthma, I had a lot of conversations with God. I promised God that I would never eat junk food again, that I'd lose fifty pounds and keep it off, that I'd even go to church if only I could be healthy again. For a few days I actually believed that maybe God had cured me. But then I had a terrible attack at three A.M. and ended up in the emergency room, and I knew this was for keeps.

—Kim, age forty-one

The bargaining stage is usually the last, futile effort to find a way out of having to accept a hidden disability. You may make bargains with yourself, with your family, with God, even with the Devil—anyone who might be able to make you feel better again. Since neither denial nor anger worked in ridding yourself of this affliction, you hope for a miracle of some sort.

When Elisabeth Kubler-Ross conceptualized the bargaining stage, she wasn't conveying a disrespect toward religious beliefs and prayer. For many, daily prayer is comforting, and a belief in a Higher Power can offer hope. Bargaining is different than normal prayer: It is about desperately trying to eliminate your hidden disability by promising to change your life in exchange for good health.

Bargaining is similar to the childhood stage of "magical thinking." If children wish that their parents would come home early from work and they do, the children may believe that their thoughts caused this to happen. As the children get older, they realize that their thoughts can't control their world. Yet, as an adult who's developed a hidden disability, your inner child reemerges. By making promises to do or not to do something, you secretly believe you'll recover.

Bargaining is usually a short, transitory stage. After making bargains doesn't work, the illusion fades. You still have a hidden disability even though you've vowed to be a better person. When the miracle of recovery fails to occur, you may then succumb to the next stage of grief: depression.

Stage Four: Depression

After the denial has worn off and the anger has dissipated, it's common to sink into a period of depression. Depression is different than sadness. Sadness comes and goes; often just by acknowledging that you're sad and perhaps crying a bit, you feel relief. Depression is deeper, more profound, and potentially more destructive than sadness.

Like clouds on an overcast day, depression doesn't easily lift. When you're depressed, you lose your ability to enjoy a beautiful sunrise, the presence of loved ones, a favorite song. You might stare off into space, feeling distracted, or even lose and forget things more often. You may long for the past and fear the future. Engaging in unhealthy activities, such as drugs, alcohol, eating disorders, reckless driving, or unsafe sex, may also be signs of depression. You may even find yourself seriously contemplating suicide.

Signs of Depression

According to the *Diagnostic and Statistical Manual IV* (*DSM IV*) (American Psychiatric Association 1994), you're suffering from a major depression if you have five or more of the following symptoms during a two-week period:

1. Depressed mood each day

2. Lack of interest or pleasure

3. Significant weight loss or gain

4. Insomnia or sleeping too much

5. Being either agitated or lethargic

6. Fatigued; no energy

7. Feeling worthlessness and inappropriate guilt

8. Trouble concentrating or indecisiveness

9. Recurrent thoughts of suicide

Types of Depression

There are two major types of depression—endogenous and exogenous. Someone suffering from "endogenous depression" has been depressed much of his or her life, often with no clear trigger. He or she is blue even when life is going well. Resulting from a biochemical imbalance, this type of depression is, in and of itself, a hidden disability.

The other type, "exogenous depression" is strikingly different. Your depression results from a crisis—such as a divorce, death, job loss, financial ruin, or fire. In time, your depression lifts as you adjust to new circumstances. A hidden disability can cause this type of depression. Given that your symptoms wax and wane, your depression may come and go as well. When you're having a flare-up, you may feel depressed, but once you feel better, your depression dissipates. Feeling depressed is an understandable reaction to being in physical discomfort, especially with a disability that is doubted and disqualified.

The depression of a hidden disability is often misunderstood by others. Some people declare that depression causes hidden disabilities. All you need to do, the argument goes, is treat your depression and your physical problems will disappear. While some people are depressed prior to becoming disabled, it's simplistic to assert that depression is at the root of physical problems. Most people with hidden disabilities feel that they would no longer be depressed if their health condition vanished. In contrast, someone with endogenous depression would remain depressed. And, while antidepressants are often used to treat pain, this doesn't mean that hidden disabilities are psychosomatic. Both depression and chronic pain deplete chemicals in the brain that antidepressants restore.

Understanding Your Depression

Hilary, who's had chronic fatigue syndrome for seven years, thinks about suicide daily. Her CFIDS is severe; she can barely get out of bed, has seizures, and is debilitated by joint pains. After depleting her life savings on treatments, nothing has helped. Many of Hilary's friends, who were once supportive, have stopped calling.

June, who's had myofascial pain syndrome for a year, felt depressed when first diagnosed. But regular chiropractic treatments, physical therapy, and daily walks have greatly alleviated her pain and her depression. She also counts on the loving support of her partner and friends.

The fact that Hilary is more depressed is no coincidence; her severe and relentless symptoms are enormously hard to bear. She has little social support and feels abandoned by others. In contrast, June's pain is manageable. She's found healers who have helped. She also has the emotional and financial support of loved ones.

Whether your depression is mild or severe may depend in part on your life circumstances. Ask yourself the following questions to understand the depth and extent of your depression:

1. What's the severity or gravity of your hidden disability? If your hidden disability is manageable, like June's, your depression may also be mild. If you resemble Hilary, you're more likely to be seriously depressed. Disabilities that progress, have sudden and severe flare-ups, or involve several parts of the body are often extremely depressing.

2. What was your emotional state before your hidden disability? If you were unhappy with your life before you became ill, it may be harder for the depression to abate.

3. What's your personality style? If you're highly anxious and prone to catastrophizing, you'll be overwhelmed by the unpredictable nature of your hidden disability. Calm and unflappable people might adapt more easily.

4. What's your social support like? Having nurturing people in your life will make your plight easier to bear. If people around you are unsupportive, your depression may persist.

5. What's the nature of your pain? Constant, unrelenting pain and/or fatigue may produce feelings of helplessness and despair that lead to suicidal thoughts.

6. What are the other stressors in your life? If you're also dealing with relationship, child, money, and/or job difficulties, you're overwhelmed and thus vulnerable to depression.

7. Were you recently diagnosed? Being depressed soon after being diagnosed may be natural. However, still being depressed six months later indicates a more significant problem.

8. Does your depression follow any pattern? For instance, if you're depressed when you have a flare-up and not depressed when it ceases, you may be having an understandable reaction to the pain and anxiety of a flare-up.

9. Are you thinking about suicide? Thoughts of suicide indicate serious depression; they should always be taken seriously, and professional help should be sought.

10. Is your depression interfering with your daily life, such as working, doing housework, or even sleeping and eating? If you can barely function due to your depression, then it's time to seek help.

Serious Depression

If you are in the midst of a serious depression, you may be barely functioning and thus seeing suicide as a viable option. In fact, you may be preoccupied with thoughts of dying—believing that this is your only escape. Your friends and family are concerned and may have urged you to seek help. (Read the following list to see whether you're at risk for a suicide attempt. If so, you should seek professional help immediately.)

Symptoms of Suicide Risk:

- Having a plan in mind for how to carry out the suicide

- Feeling hopeless and despairing, as though there's nothing to live for

- Giving away personal belongings

- Making a will and/or buying an insurance plan

- Having access to the means to commit suicide, such as possessing firearms, pills, knives

- Talking about suicide to others

- Living alone and having few friends

- A prior suicide attempt

- A family history of suicide and/or having a close friend commit suicide

- Alcohol and drug abuse

- Sudden unexplained high after a depressed period

- Being diagnosed with endogenous depression or bipolar disorder

None of these factors alone may predict a suicide attempt. Obviously people live alone and do fine, and it's common to buy an insurance plan. Also, paradoxically, sometimes knowing that suicide is an option may be comforting for you. You have the security of knowing you could escape your pain—even though you vow never to attempt it. However, statistically, these factors do place you at higher risk for a suicide attempt.

What Do You Do if You're at Risk for Suicide?

- See a seasoned mental health professional knowledgeable about the depression of chronic illness and pain.

- Consider medication. A medical doctor can prescribe antidepressants to help you get a handle on your depression.

- If you're seriously considering suicide, a short stay in a psychiatric hospital may be necessary. There's no need to feel badly about this; it's just a way to get the help you need.

- Join a support group that focuses on your disability or on more general topics such as pain.

- Make a list of all you have to live for. Include the people in your life you love. Describe how each of these people would be affected by your suicide. Remind yourself how devastated they'd be.

- Recall the times that you have felt better. Keep a journal to remind yourself that your mood and pain level do improve at times.

- Call a sympathetic friend and confide your feelings.

- If you're religious, speak to your clergy person. Prayer or meditation may help.

- Recall how you've dealt with a difficult situation before. Write down the strengths that helped you to cope. Remember that those same strengths are within you now.

- Call a suicide prevention hot line to talk.

- Remember that suicide is a permanent solution to a temporary state of mind.

Other Ways to Relieve Depression

Even if you are not seriously depressed, you may want to restore a sense of purpose and joy to your life. Here are some ways to feel better:

- Help others. Depression makes you self-preoccupied. The gratification of helping another may improve your mood.

- Be with optimistic people. Depression is contagious. Try to spend time with upbeat people who are coping well with life.

- Speak to the people in your life who are critical and unsupportive. Let them know the impact on you. If this doesn't work, avoid them and replace them with more compassionate, supportive people.

- Notice your posture. Are you slouched? Do you hold your head down? Sometimes simply sitting upright with your head held high can make you feel better.

- Focus on what you can do, not on what you can't. If you used to run but now can only walk a couple of blocks, try to enjoy the walk. Notice what's beautiful and special all around you.

- Remember that you're not alone. Millions of other people are struggling with a hidden disability and most feel depressed from time to time. Chances are that your depressed mood will lift at some point.

Stage Five: Acceptance

The final stage of grieving is acceptance. Kubler-Ross imagined this stage to be a peaceful one, when the struggles of depression and anger have subsided. You realize that your loss is permanent and your life has been changed irrevocably. You accept your predicament and live well in the present.

Yet with a hidden disability, acceptance isn't so easy. You may come to accept your back pain only to find your pain traveling to your neck and shoulders. You accept your limited lifestyle only to have a resurgence of symptoms and consequently new losses. Since your symptoms may be constantly changing, your emotions switch back and forth, from acceptance, to anger, to depression, than back to acceptance. Understandably, you're more tolerant when your symptoms are mild; then you descend into despair when you've flared up.

While you may not be able to totally accept your hidden disability, you can embrace your life as it is. This means accepting yourself as a valuable, although flawed, human being. You are not just your hidden disability. If instead you long for a different body or someone else's life, you'll despair. Rejecting who you are leaves you feeling deficient and helpless. Acceptance also means appreciating what is working in your life. While you can easily recount the frustrations and losses, acceptance involves seeing the total picture—the people who love you, the simple pleasures of being alive, the parts of your body that do work.

Working toward Acceptance

If you continue to deny your hidden disability, figure out why you're fighting acceptance. Some of the reasons may be based on your particular type of health problem. There also may be personal obstacles standing in the way. Take a moment to answer the following questions.

1. My symptoms fluctuate. ____ *Yes* ____ *No*

2. Few health care professionals understand how to help my condition.
____ *Yes* ____ *No*

3. My hidden disability is progressive or life threatening.
____ *Yes* ____ *No*

4. I have no definite diagnosis. ____ *Yes* ____ *No*

5. I'm at risk of developing a more serious problem. ____ *Yes* ____ *No*

6. I'm in a great deal of pain. ____ *Yes* ____ *No*

7. I'm exhausted most of the time. ____ *Yes* ____ *No*

8. I can hardly function at home and work. ____ *Yes* ____ *No*

9. I have little hope that I'll ever improve. ____ *Yes* ____ *No*

If you've answered "yes" to any of these questions, no wonder it's hard to completely accept your disability. It's a struggle to accept a medical condition that is frightening, painful, and unstable. There may also be personal roadblocks in your way. Answer the following questions to see what else may be getting in the way.

1. If I truly accepted my hidden disability, what would I need to give up?

   _____

   _____

2. What would be good about accepting my hidden disability? _____

   _____

   _____

3. What would be negative about accepting my hidden disability? _____

   _____

   _____

4. Who else in my life is having trouble accepting my hidden disability? ____

   _____

   _____

5. Would this person or these people have difficulty if I truly accepted my hidden disability? _____

   _____

6. Now review your answers. What do you learn from them? _____

   _____

   _____

When she answered these questions, Fran, a forty-seven-year-old woman with fibromyalgia, was surprised at her response to the question about what she'd have to give up; she answered "hope." By accepting her fibromyalgia, she was giving up the chance of recovery. She explains:

> I know this sounds crazy, but somehow I always felt that to get better I'd need this macho attitude, like "I'm going to beat this thing." I guess this comes from my father who never admitted when he was in pain or sick. He'd go to work with the flu. I remember him hobbling off to a business meeting with a sprained ankle.

From these childhood experiences, Fran assumed that by accepting her disability, she was admitting defeat. As long as she resisted the diagnosis, it didn't really exist. Deep down she feared that acceptance meant hopelessness. While perseverance and faith can be essential tools to fight any illness, Fran's macho attitude led to workaholism, over-committing herself socially, and ignoring early warning signs of a flare-up. She realized that she could accept her illness without giving up her fighting spirit.

The Impact of Others on Acceptance

When Peter, a forty-two-year-old man recently diagnosed with diabetes, answered these questions, he made a remarkable discovery: He wasn't having such a hard time accepting his illness, but his wife and son were. His wife admonished him to lose weight and blamed his diabetes on his extra fifteen pounds. His teenage son teased him about being a couch potato. Neither wanted to believe that Peter had developed a potentially serious, chronic illness that jeopardized their stability. Thus, if Peter accepted his illness, he'd be alienating himself from his family.

Your loved ones may be loath to accept the hidden disability that has become an unwanted part of family life. They deny your problem for various reasons, for example, to distance themselves for their own fears of illness or because of their considerable anxiety about you. If the reactions of others are getting in the way of your own acceptance, speak to them. Let them know how their denial and resistance are affecting you, and work with them toward improved communication and understanding.

Tools for Accepting a Hidden Disability

Here are some tools to help you better accept your hidden disability:

- Acceptance doesn't mean giving up! You can accept that, at this moment, you have a particular condition. Yet you can remain hopeful that your hidden disability may eventually get better or become more tolerable. At the same time, it's important to own the disability as yours. While you didn't ask for this problem, a hidden disability has become part of your life.

- Remind yourself, "I have a disability. I am not my disability. I am more than the sum of my health problems. I have talents, interests, and strengths aside from my physical condition."

- Connect with others who are living well with a hidden disability. Check out support groups or chat rooms on the Internet.

- Give yourself an assignment to truly accept your hidden disability for a limited amount of time. For instance, say, "I'll accept my disability for just one hour." See what feelings come up when you try this for a short period.

- Recognize that feelings of acceptance may come and go. Don't berate yourself if you are again denying your hidden disability.

Reminders

Grief is a natural process when you develop a hidden disability.

Grief is circular, not linear. You may feel angry, then accepting, then angry again.

While anger is a normal emotion that comes and goes, bitterness and hostility are toxic to you and others. Find ways to work with anger so it doesn't turn hostile.

Feelings of depression may come and go. But if you feel debilitated by depression, and especially if you feel suicidal, you must seek help.

You can come to accept your hidden disability without giving up your hope or fighting spirit.

Know that acceptance also comes and goes. Try not to beat up on yourself if you haven't "resolved" your grief.

CHAPTER 3

Dealing with
Difficult Emotions

When I got the flu, I didn't worry—at least at first. But after three weeks passed, I couldn't figure out why this thing wouldn't go away. So I started going to doctors and then more doctors. Weeks passed, I had so many tests, and yet no one knew what was wrong. When I was still sick six months later, I was beside myself. Terrified, angry, depressed. I worried about my job. I felt guilty because I couldn't help much with the house or the kids. I felt ashamed to be bedridden with an illness that had no diagnosis. One day, I was reading about chronic fatigue syndrome in a woman's magazine. It all fit! They were describing me. Suddenly my illness had a name. I was thrilled!

—Kate, age thirty-nine

The effect of having a hidden disability is far-reaching; it influences your biological, psychological, social, and spiritual/existential worlds. Kate's story illustrates the many feelings that accompany a hidden disability. You feel sad, angry, scared—sometimes all in the same day or even the same hour. You're also excited or hopeful when a problem is finally diagnosed or when a flare-up ceases.

There are many factors at work here. First there are biological and physical realities: Being ill is depressing. Chronic pain causes irritability, helplessness, and despair. Feeling exhausted most of the time is frustrating. Some medications may make you even more depressed and anxious. And with some disorders—low thyroid, for instance—depression is a common symptom.

Then there's the psychological toll of being sick or disabled. Being derailed from your career path and your hobbies is depressing. No longer being able to be a jogger, a painter, or whatever it was that you once identified yourself as being, hurts your pride. Hearing about a friend's ski trip or a cousin's promotion may fill you with envy and self-pity. And when despite your best efforts—the trips to the doctors, the thousands of dollars on various treatments, the special diets and vitamins—you still have a hidden disability, you become angry.

Along with the psychological, there's the social aspect. First, many people don't recognize that you have a hidden disability. It's aggravating to continually have to convince people that your disability is real. Also, since the culture tends to deny illness and disability, others become threatened by your fragile state. To avoid dealing with their own vulnerability to illness, they withdraw. Or, feeling out of place, you distance yourself.

Lastly, there's the spiritual/existential component of having a hidden disability. When you're healthy it's easy to believe that you'll always live a healthy life. A hidden disability shatters this belief. Now you're confronted with harsh realities: Health problems are common and sometimes unavoidable, and you are mortal.

You may start questioning all of your beliefs: Is there really a God? If so, why would God let this happen to me? How can I be truly happy knowing that there's so much in life (like my hidden disability) that I can't control? Developing a hidden disability shakes the very foundation of your life.

Given the enormous impact of your disability on every part of your life, it's no wonder that you feel intense emotions at times. This chapter will describe some of the most common emotions. We've already talked about depression and anger. But there are many other emotions you contend with, such as helplessness, envy, and self-pity. While these feelings are unavoidable, there are skills you can develop for coping.

Common Emotions

Fear and Anxiety

I'm afraid all the time. When I wake up, I feel scared to get out of bed and face another day. I'm scared of falling and hurting myself. I'm scared of the future. I'm worried about being a burden to my family. I can't even get any peace when I sleep because I have nightmares and wake up all tense and agitated.

—Naomi, age 45, recently
diagnosed with multiple sclerosis

When you're stricken with an ailment that wrecks havoc with your life, you become afraid. The fear stems from feeling out of control, from not knowing what the future will bring. Physiologically, fear produces stress hormones that in turn create tension and a heightened sensitivity. Since biologically we're still animals, humans respond to danger with a primitive "fight-or-flight" response. Thus, physically as well as emotionally, our bodies go on high alert; we may misinterpret external cues as dangerous; and our muscles are tight and poised to escape or attack.

The list of fears related to having a hidden disability are long. In fact, when we're afraid, our mind can create an unlimited number of worries. Some of the more common fears are listed below. Check off those you've felt in the last month.

Body Fears

_____ A recurrence/relapse

_____ Developing new symptoms

_____ Becoming unattractive

_____ Becoming too fat or too skinny

_____ Hurting yourself through activity

_____ Hurting yourself through inactivity

_____ Dying

_____ Developing a more serious disease

_____ Losing capacities (e.g., bladder control, ability to walk, hearing)

_____ The consequences of wrong medical treatment

_____ The consequences of not choosing treatment

_____ Medication side effects

_____ Having to have surgery

_____ Pain worsening

_____ Other body fears: _____

_____

Rejection Fears

_____ Losing friends

_____ Losing your significant other

_____ Not being able to find a significant other

_____ Losing family members

_____ Losing your job

_____ Losing your children's love

_____ Other rejection fears: _____

Hidden Disability Fears

_____ People not understanding what you're going through

_____ People ridiculing you for your symptoms

_____ Your doctors not taking your concerns seriously

_____ Your boss not accommodating your special needs

_____ Not being able to ask for what you need because your disability is hidden

_____ Other hidden disability fears: _____

Other Fears

_____ Money problems

_____ Burdening others

_____ Losing control over your life

_____ Fear of sleeping

_____ Fear of eating

_____ Your significant other and/or children becoming ill

_____ Missing out on opportunities

_____ Other fears: _____

If you've checked off a number of fears, fear is definitely impacting your life. Are you particularly worried about rejection from others? Are most of your fears around advocating for your special needs? If you've checked fears in numerous areas, this may suggest that your fear is pervasive in your life. Many people who experience this pervasive fear fall under the diagnosis of having generalized anxiety disorder (GAD). While it's valuable to see what's causing the fear, the next step is to manage it. Fear left unchecked may turn into anxiety or even panic.

Anxiety and Panic Attacks

Anxiety is generalized fear. While fear is focused on a particular experience, such as fear of going bankrupt, anxiety has no bounds. Anxiety creates an ominous sense of dread that something bad will happen at any moment. Thus, anxious people have nervous stomachs, tight muscles, and high-strung temperaments because they're perpetually braced for disaster to strike.

Naomi, the woman with multiple sclerosis whose words opened this chapter, explains her anxiety this way:

> I've always been a nervous person, but I'm much worse since my diagnosis. Everything scares me. Even though my symptoms are still mild and hardly affect my life, I'm just waiting to get sicker. I went to a support group and there was a woman there in a wheelchair. Now I'm consumed with fear about ending up like her. My husband is losing his patience with me. I don't know how much more he can take. I just can't help it. It's like my worries have a mind of their own.

Naomi's understandable fears of her illness have snowballed into generalized anxiety disorder. Anxiety is making her life unmanageable, ironically more so than her physical symptoms. Naomi needs to learn to cope with her anxiety, since her endless worrying is doing nothing to help her disease and may even exacerbate her symptoms.

If Naomi's anxiety continues to grow, she may develop panic attacks, which are intense states of terror that occur unpredictably. They're called "panic attacks" because you literally feel like you're being attacked, and your body becomes flooded with stress hormones. During a panic attack, your body launches a full-blown defensive assault causing symptoms such as heart palpitations, trembling, shaking, sweating, flushing, chest pains, shortness of breath, dizziness, and/or nausea. Because of the intense and frightening physical symptoms, you may feel that you are going to pass out, even die. And yet physically there's nothing wrong: it's merely panic.

Sheryl, a nurse with diabetes, describes a panic attack she experienced:

> I was seeing a patient in the emergency room for a broken finger, when all of a sudden my heart started beating so fast I thought I'd have a heart attack. I tried to ignore the symptoms and listen to the patient, but then I felt like I couldn't breathe. I had to run outside to get some air. A doctor came out after me. He knows I'm diabetic, so he checked me out thoroughly and said I was fine. He said he thought I was having a panic attack.
>
> I was shocked to hear this. I'd never had a panic attack in my life. I prided myself on being a stoic, tough kind of nurse who'd seen it all. It wasn't until later that I realized that I'd been stuffing all my feelings about being a diabetic. For some reason they all erupted at once. Maybe it was the accumulation of seeing sick and dying patients all day. My defenses collapsed.

Along with GAD and panic attacks, the following sections discuss some other anxiety disorders.

Agoraphobia

Agoraphobia is the avoidance of places or situations because of fear that you can't escape. In severe cases, a person may be unable to leave the house. Agoraphobia can develop as a result of a hidden disability because you fear others' ridicule or doubt, or because you're afraid your symptoms will worsen if you leave the house.

Phobias

Phobias are the fear and avoidance of a particular stimuli (e.g., flying, spiders, needles). As a chronically ill person, you may develop a fear of your own body, becoming phobic about seeing doctors or about taking any kind of medication. Such a phobia may impede your ability to make reasonable and informed decisions about your health care. Or you can become exercise phobic—apprehensive that any type of exertion will spark a relapse.

Obsessive-Compulsive Disorder (OCD)

Obsessions are distressing thoughts or images that you just can't shake (e.g., catching germs, dying). Compulsions are nonfunctional behavior that you feel driven to do (e.g., washing your hands over and over).

Obsessive-compulsive behavior can easily result from having a hidden disability. When you're sick, you obsess about every aspect of your body, for instance, whether you should undergo a particular medical test or try a new medication. You may become compulsive about ridding your house of possible germs or about doing your stretches as carefully as possible. While common, becoming obsessed with your illness can alienate others, agitate your mind, and cause insomnia.

Post-Traumatic Stress Disorder (PTSD)

PTSD is a term that's used to describe people who have experienced trauma (e.g., being a victim of a crime, being caught in a natural disaster, fighting in combat). The traumatized person has flashbacks of the incident, sleep problems, difficulty concentrating, hyperalertness, and/or a fear of certain people or places.

Many people with a hidden disability fit the criteria for PTSD. It's traumatic to have a hidden disability with puzzling and unpredictable symptoms that others invalidate. Other traumatic events might have occurred: surgeries, misdiagnoses, relapses, or new symptoms out of the blue; side effects from medication; or changes in physical appearance. Unremitting pain is traumatic in and of itself. While health professionals have been slow to acknowledge the relationship between chronic illness and PTSD, we believe that the trauma of a hidden disability rivals that of other calamities.

Managing Anxiety and Panic

There are several things you can do to manage fear and anxiety. And while it may be tempting to try and ignore your fears, fear left unattended will intensify. After a while, fear takes on a life of its own and turns into anxiety or panic. While it's frightening to live with a hidden disability, fear doesn't have to dominate your life. The following sections discuss effective coping skills.

Stopping the Cycle

Like a snowball rolling down a hill, fear will grow in size if you let it. By allowing fear to have free reign over your mind and ruminating over worst-case scenarios, fear will rule your life. Here's how to interrupt the cycle:

Step 1: When you notice that you're afraid or anxious, yell "Stop!" in your mind and imagine a stop sign or a red light.

Step 2: Sit down (if possible) and take three deep breaths.

Step 3: At the same time, say to yourself, "Calm ... calm ... calm," while breathing. Add a few more words that you find relaxing, such as, "It's going to be okay," "It's nothing serious, just anxiety."

Step 4: After you've reduced your anxiety, challenge negative thoughts. Say, "There's no way to predict that something bad will happen."

Step 5: If necessary, repeat steps 2 and 3.

Step 6: Distract yourself by taking a walk, playing with your pet, calling a friend, etc.

Thinking Positively

Numerous studies have demonstrated the power of both positive and negative thinking. Saying to yourself, "I'm weak," creates a downtrodden reaction. In contrast, saying, "I'm strong," increases confidence. When you become fearful, say to yourself, "I'm strong. I can handle this." For instance, if you're worried that your partner will leave you, say, "No matter what happens in my life, I am strong and can handle it."

Visualizing Positive Images

Create a soothing image that you can bring to mind whenever you are afraid, for instance, a favorite beach, the face of a beloved friend or pet, or a flower.

Repeating Positive Words

Think of a few comforting words (e.g., peace, calm, God, love, etc.) or reassuring phrases (e.g., It will be okay.) Say these words and phrases silently when you're anxious.

Remembering That Fearful Moments Will Not Last

When you feel fear, it seems like it will never go away. Remind yourself that every experience in life comes and goes—both happy and unhappy ones. No one remains in the dentist's chair forever, although it may seem that way! Remind yourself that "this too shall pass."

Realizing That Worries Don't Generally Come True

Mark Twain said it best, "I am an old man and have known a great many troubles, but most of them never happened." Most of your worries won't come true. And worrying won't have any effect on the future anyway.

Seeking Professional Help

If you have PTSD, OCD, or severe panic attacks, or if your anxiety cannot be controlled using these methods, see a licensed psychotherapist experienced in both anxiety and chronic pain and illness (see chapter 12 for information about seeking therapy).

If your anxiety or panic cannot be controlled through therapy and self-help methods, consult a psychiatrist for medication evaluation. The medications most often used for anxiety are: BuSpar; selective serotonin reuptake inhibitors (SSRI), such as Prozac, Zoloft, or Paxil; or Anafranil (for OCD) or Tofranil, which are called "tricyclic antidepressants." These medications can be used for long periods of time and are not considered physically addictive, although you may develop a psychological dependence. Like all medications, they may have side effects. Taper off any drug slowly with professional assistance.

If your doctor prescribes a class of tranquilizers called a benzodiazepine (for instance, Atavin, Valium, Xanax, or Klonopin), note that these are addictive drugs that can cause depression. Be careful about starting these drugs and, if you decide to stop them, withdraw from them slowly and only with a doctor's supervision.

Shame

I feel ashamed to tell people that I have multiple chemical sensitivities syndrome. Most people think it's all in my head. One supposed friend told me to just relax and take a vacation and I'd be fine. No one seems to understand. I feel embarrassed to always ask people about whether they have carpets or pets or if they use chemicals before going over to their house. I don't want people to think I'm nuts. But maybe I am nuts!

—Emma, age twenty-seven

In a world that expects people to be healthy, having a hidden disability evokes enormous shame and embarrassment. Embarrassment refers to a momentary reaction to something that's happened, for example, having to ask for a special chair or having to lie down at a party. Shame is a deeper and potentially more destructive emotion. The core of shame is believing that you're bad, deficient, unworthy. When you feel ashamed, your "badness" is being exposed to the world.

Emma believes that exposing her injured and disabled self will cause others to condemn or ridicule her. And, unfortunately, she's had that experience more than once. When people question her symptoms, she feels even more ashamed and starts doubting her own sanity. This only makes her want to hide from the world.

To see the role that shame plays in your life, check off the following statements that apply to you.

Since developing my hidden disability, I feel ashamed of:

_____ my appearance

_____ having to ask for special accommodations

_____ telling people about my condition

_____ meeting new people

_____ feeling different from others

_____ doing less around the house

_____ working less than others

_____ being ill and/or in pain

_____ being sexual

_____ other shameful experiences: _____

If you checked several of the above, shame is affecting your life on a daily basis and is undermining your self-confidence. You may hide from others to avoid scrutiny. If you were raised in a dysfunctional family with substance abuse, child abuse, and/or domestic violence, you're more vulnerable to feeling shame. Also, if a parent used shame to control and discipline (e.g., "You're a bad girl/boy," "You're stupid," "What's the matter with you?"), you might have always grappled with shame.

Shame, like anxiety, can be diminished through practice. Following are some techniques to try.

Expanding Awareness

Notice when you feel shame (nonverbal cues might include blushing, slouching your shoulders, or avoiding eye contact). Then, take several deep breaths while repeating to yourself, "I'm a good person. I have nothing to feel ashamed about. It's not my fault that I have a hidden disability."

Recalling Childhood Memories

If you've lived with a lot of shame during your life, recall a childhood incident where you were shamed (for instance, your parent yelling, "You'll never amount to anything!"). Remind yourself that the seeds of shame were planted years ago. You may even have a mental "tape" replaying in your head from past shameful experiences. Now a hidden disability may be intensifying shame. Yet you have the power to challenge and refute the negative things that people have said about you. Repeat to yourself, "Shame is an old 'tape' in my life. But I have nothing to be ashamed of."

Using Symbols

Create a symbol that represents your feelings of shame. For instance, Emma envisioned an injured puppy cowering in the corner. Now expand your vision to include someone or something comforting this shamed part. Emma imagined a female Great Dane protecting and nurturing the injured puppy.

Guilt

I feel guilty for developing this back problem because I'm such a burden to my husband. He works all day, then he has to help me with the cooking, the kids, and the house when he gets home. Weekends he does all the laundry and the shopping. And what do I do? Lie around on ice packs and take Vicodin.

—Cynthia, age forty, diagnosed
with a herniated disc

Some people equate shame with guilt, but they're actually very different emotions. Shame is an all-encompassing experience of yourself as defective and bad. Guilt is feeling bad about an action you did or didn't do. In other words, when you feel guilty, you believe you *did* something bad. When you're ashamed, you feel that you *are* bad.

Not all guilt is irrational. "Healthy guilt" occurs when you violate your moral values. If you cheat on your taxes or your significant other, "forget" to return your neighbor's tools, or drink and drive, you feel guilty for good reasons. This "healthy guilt" prods you to act more responsibly.

Some of your guilt about your hidden disability may also be the healthy kind. For instance, if Cynthia, with the herniated disc, becomes significantly overweight, her guilt communicates that she's jeopardizing her health. But much of the guilt associated with a hidden disability is harmful and self-defeating. Cynthia's feeling guilty for being disabled only makes her suffer for something that isn't her fault. She ends up feeling like an inadequate spouse and mother, without recognizing her own value. This type of guilt fosters self-loathing and feelings of failure.

Use the following exercise to see whether your guilty feelings are "healthy" or "unhealthy."

Healthy Guilt

I feel guilty because:

_____ I eat poorly.

_____ I forget to take my medications.

_____ I don't do my exercises.

_____ I push myself more than I should.

_____ I do things that are risky, for example, drinking, drugs, overeating, and/or having unsafe sex.

_____ I overwork.

_____ I can never say "no."

_____ I complain all the time.

_____ I lash out at others.

Unhealthy Guilt

I feel guilty because:

_____ I'm sick a lot.

_____ I'm tired a lot.

_____ I don't do as much as I should around the house.

_____ I don't feel as sexual as I'd like to.

_____ I don't help with the kids as much.

_____ I'm not earning as much money as I should.

_____ I'm not saving money like I should.

_____ I'm moody.

_____ I'm not as happy and cheerful as I used to be.

_____ I don't do as much household tasks as I should.

_____ Others do more for me than I do for them.

If you are checking a lot of examples of "healthy guilty," your guilt can motivate you to take better care of yourself. Think of your guilt as a wake-up call to pay more attention to your needs. It's an urgent message from your more responsible self. But if you mostly checked "unhealthy guilt," then your task is different—it's to challenge these negative and harmful beliefs. Berating yourself and feeling guilty for having a hidden disability serve no useful purpose, can exacerbate your symptoms, and can severely hurt your relationships with yourself and others.

Following are some ways to reduce unhealthy guilt.

Using Thought-Stopping Techniques

Stop the thoughts and confront these unhelpful judgments. Say, "I have nothing to feel guilty about. I didn't choose to have a hidden disability. I'm still a worthwhile and good person."

Battling Guilt

Imagine yourself in a battle with guilt. Challenge your opponent just as you would a threatening aggressor. Tell guilt, "I won't let you control my life. I won't let you in. I have no use for you."

Recognizing Your Efforts

Make a list of all the ways you have tried to manage having a hidden disability (for example, drinking lots of water, spending money on different health care practitioners, reading books). Keep this list on hand and read it when you feel guilty. Remind yourself how hard you've been trying.

Envy

Last Sunday, I was having a pretty good day. I went out and walked a couple of blocks and sat in the park. I was just soaking up the sunshine when I saw a friend. She was rollerblading with her boyfriend. Instantly my good mood became black. I felt so envious of her good health, all the fun they were having. Suddenly my being able to walk two blocks seemed pathetic.

—Maggie, age twenty-eight,
who has rheumatoid arthritis

Envy is one of the most common and painful of emotions. You may envy others' good health, their freedom of mobility, their ability to work ten-hour days and travel around the world. While envy is understandable, when it's left to grow, it's destructive. Envy spoils a good day and makes a triumph seem insignificant. Envy damages your self-concept and debases your good efforts.

Envy also separates you from others. When you believe other people are luckier, you feel cursed. This sense of being different alienates you, contributing to loneliness. Yet the truth is that no one escapes difficulty. While you may covet another's apparent good health and happiness, this is your envy speaking. All of life's struggles—for self-esteem, security, contentment, love—are shared. Almost everyone confronts illness. Grief and loss are universal life experiences.

Even without a hidden disability, most people feel envious at times. The culture fuels envy so that new and more expensive products are consumed. A person earning $50,000 a year envies someone making $100,000. Given that envy is built into the fabric of society, the added burden of a hidden disability can make envy ever-present in your life. While it may be unavoidable to occasionally feel envious, don't let it dominate your life. Persistent envy will sabotage your efforts.

Use the following exercise to gauge whether you feel envy on a regular or occasional basis (circle one):

1. I envy my friends' good health.
              Daily   *Occasionally*   *Never*

2. I envy other people's freedom of mobility.
              Daily   *Occasionally*   *Never*

3. I envy other people's physical appearance.
              Daily   *Occasionally*   *Never*

4. My efforts seem minuscule compared to what other people are accomplishing.
              Daily   *Occasionally*   *Never*

5. I wish I could become someone else.
              Daily   *Occasionally*   *Never*

Review your answers. If you've feeling envious on a daily basis, you're discouraged and minimizing your successes. The following sections offer some ways to counteract envy.

Avoid Assumptions

Don't assume that you're the only one struggling with health problems; you might be surprised by what other people are facing. Your disability is hidden, and theirs might be as well. Maggie, a therapist-in-training with arthritis, learned this lesson firsthand:

> I was taking a weekend class and feeling really flared-up. My joints were killing me. There was this one woman in the class who just seemed the picture of good health: rosy cheeks, athletic build, and a really friendly, outgoing disposition. I envied her so much. Well, wouldn't you know it, I got paired up with her for an exercise! One person was the client and the other the counselor; then we switched roles. I started telling her how exhausted I felt, how my joints ached. She was warm and sensitive which was nice, but I still resented her since I didn't believe she could really understand what I was going through. When we switched roles, I was just astonished when she told me that she had been diagnosed with cancer last month and was considering her options! My jaw dropped; I was speechless. And I felt so ashamed of myself for resenting her.

Even if a person is healthy, they're likely coping with some adversity. They may be confronting a family or relationship problem, poor self-esteem, or childhood traumas that haunt them. The point is that life can be hard, and everyone has his or her share of suffering as well as joy.

Practice "Mudita"

Try to cultivate "mudita," which is a Buddhist term for "sympathetic joy." Buddhists believe that all people are connected, and therefore joyous events for one person are shared by all. Therefore, someone's else's good health or success can be viewed as benefiting everyone.

Self-Pity

One of my friends told me the other day that I feel sorry for myself too much. Well, that's easy for him to say! He doesn't have to live with carpal tunnel syndrome. He's not on medical disability, he doesn't have to ask his wife to drive him around. You bet I feel sorry for myself!

—Greg, age forty-one

When you have a hidden disability, it's common to feel self-pity. You lament your physical suffering and your constricted life. You hone in on your losses and disappointments. You wonder whether you're somehow cursed. Feeling sorry for yourself is, at times, unavoidable, especially when you're flared up and have to cancel plans. However, try not to indulge in self-pity. If you do, you'll feel defeated and dejected. Self-pity also produces an intense self-focus that causes you to miss out on the positive aspects of your life.

Like with envy, self-pity isolates you from others. You feel unique in your suffering. Consequently, others may avoid you, which only reinforces your feelings of being different. Again, remember that life is hard for everyone at times. The enormously popular book, *The Road Less Traveled*, begins, "Life is difficult" (Peck 1997). Millions of people from around the world have been drawn to this book because Peck's words capture their experience. One way to combat self-pity is to remember that you're not alone in facing hardship.

To counteract self-pity, it also helps to evaluate its pervasiveness in your life. How often do you feel self-pity? Check any statements you agree with.

_____ I'm a loser.

_____ I hate my life.

_____ I have it worse than most people.

_____ It's just not fair.

_____ Why did this have to happen to me?

_____ Even God has stopped caring about me.

_____ Nobody loves me.

_____ I'm a hopeless case.

_____ My life sucks.

_____ Why me?

If you checked any of these statements, self-pity may be a negative force in your life. The following sections offer some ways to reduce self-pity.

Appreciate What You Do Have

What distinguishes a happy person from a miserable one is often not life circumstances—it's attitude. By appreciating what you do have, you feel better. Focusing on your losses generates unhappiness.

Act "As If" You Aren't Feeling Self-Pity

By acting as though you are grateful, even when you're mired in self-pity, you can affect a great change in your feelings over time. While at first glance this approach may seem dishonest, remember that how you act can influence and alter your mood. Experiments have shown that subjects asked to smile rated their moods as happier than those instructed to frown.

Try your own experiment. When you're feeling sorry for yourself, rate your self-pity on a scale of 1 to 5. Set the timer for twenty minutes. During this time, act as though you are appreciative of your life. Go outside and find three things to admire, such as a flower. Smile at the person across the street. Now, rate yourself again on the scale. If your envy went down even a point, you can see the power of acting more grateful.

Help Others

Possibly the best way to escape your self-scrutiny is to reach out to others. Even small acts like calling a friend in need makes you feel valuable and productive.

Powerlessness

> Since my heart attack last year, I feel like I've lost total control over my life. Before I was successful, I dated pretty much who I wanted, and I traveled around the world. Now I work intermittently, and I rarely date because I'm sometimes impotent from the medication. Anyway, I'm too nervous to have sex because I don't want to trigger another heart attack. Even though my doctor says I can exercise, I'm scared to do that, too. I feel powerless over every aspect of my life.
>
> —Les, age forty-six

Like Les, at one time, you may have had more control over the circumstances of your life. If you wanted to, you'd be able to take on virtually any task. Eating healthy foods, exercising, and thinking positively seemed to guarantee good health. Although you experienced occasional disappointments and setbacks in life, you bounced back. By working hard and persevering, you could achieve what you wanted.

Now that you've developed a hidden disability, you probably feel like you've lost all your power. Your life has been turned upside down. Even though you've tried virtually everything possible, you're still stuck with a medical problem. It's natural to believe that you must be doing something wrong. If only you stretched more (or less), ate more (or less), or found just the right treatment, you'd regain your health—and your life. You scrutinize every action to try to regain control. Yet, when your efforts don't succeed, you feel like a victim, with no ability to impact your life.

Developing a hidden disability confronts you with a painful, though universal, truth: We all have only limited control over our lives. Everyone faces disappointments, illnesses, loss, and death. While your challenges may be different than someone else's, no one has any more control. And, although you can't always influence the circumstances of your life, you can control your reactions. You can become embittered about developing a hidden disability. Or your illness can open your heart to others' suffering. You can practice self-love and forgiveness. Or you can berate yourself daily. Only you have power over your attitude.

To see the role of powerlessness in your life, check the statements with which you agree:

_____ My life is a complete mess.

_____ I can't get out of this hole I'm in.

_____ I feel trapped.

_____ I wish that someone would rescue me.

_____ I give up.

_____ I don't have the energy to keep up the fight.

_____ God has abandoned me.

_____ Nobody can help me.

_____ I can't do anything right.

_____ I feel like a victim of circumstances I can't control.

If you checked any of these statements, then powerlessness may be agitating and disheartening you. To manage powerlessness, try the suggestions in the following sections.

Letting Go

If you're a control freak, letting go will be a formidable task. You fear that by letting go you're more vulnerable to setbacks and disappointments. But holding onto the idea of control leaves you feeling like a failure every time your disability flares up. By working on letting go, you can appreciate life as it is. You don't have to change anything. You can stop working so hard at controlling reality and start living your life.

But be realistic; don't expect yourself to let go every moment of the day. Virtually no one has entirely defeated control issues. However, practicing letting go can be a great relief. Here's an exercise to try: Set a timer for five minutes. Sit comfortably and assign yourself the task of letting go of all expectations for these few minutes. Say to yourself, "For five minutes, I'll be happy just sitting here, expecting nothing. My life doesn't have to be any different than it is. I'll just appreciate the experience of being alive." You can slowly increase the time, if you find this exercise helpful.

The Serenity Prayer

The Serenity Prayer is a comforting practice when you feel out of control. Try sitting or lying in a comfortable chair, taking several deep breaths, and repeating to yourself this phrase: God grant me the serenity to accept the things I cannot change, courage to change the things I can, and wisdom to know the difference.

Emotions Can Hurt, Emotions Can Heal

To live with a hidden disability is to experience strong, overwhelming, and often frightening emotions. You're scared when you have a new symptom, then angry when a friend is unsympathetic, then joyful when a doctor offers hope. Your emotions might be so strong that they startle and alarm you. You may cry a lot even though you've never considered yourself overly emotional.

Having strong feelings when you're ill is normal. The reality is that having a hidden disability forever changes your life. The changes, however, don't all have to be for the worse. Your emotions can hurt you, but they also can heal. There may be renewed opportunities for introspection and intimacy with others. Slowing down allows you time to "smell the roses." You may reevaluate your priorities and make positive changes.

Consider David and John, two men in their thirties diagnosed with AIDS, and their different reactions to being ill. David was a self-absorbed workaholic before his diagnosis. He had a lot of friends but most were shallow, party companions. Weekends were devoted to having fun and obtaining new "toys." His biggest goal in his life was to some day buy a BMW.

When David found out he had AIDS, his illusions about his self-importance and personal power were forever shattered. Devastated and terrified, he couldn't work, and he stayed home drinking most of the day. He had what he called a "mini nervous breakdown," during which he spent a weekend crying in bed. He realized that he wasn't only crying for his lost future but about how much time he had wasted on a superficial life. He saw clearly how precious was his remaining time and became determined not to waste any of it.

His transformation amazed and impressed his friends. He sold his computer business and devoted his time to volunteering at an AIDS organization. He tutored an HIV-positive teenager. As his best friend put it, "David became a completely different person. He was a fun guy before but was really just a lightweight. But he became this caring and compassionate person that you just wanted to be around." When he died, he was surrounded by many close friends.

Contrast this to John's story. He was also a success-oriented man with few connections to others. When first diagnosed, he denied the severity of his illness and continued to work until he came down with pneumonia. He was furious at the man who had infected him. He couldn't let go of his anger and talked about it constantly. John remained bitter to the end. He spent his last year isolated and alone. Even on his deathbed, he wasn't able to forgive the man and release his animosity.

These examples show that while you can't always control the type and extent of an illness, you do have control over how you respond. You can react to your hidden disability by becoming self-absorbed and shutting down emotionally, or you can use it as a catalyst for deepening and expanding your life. Like David, you can become more compassionate and giving. The choice is yours.

Reminders

It's common to feel strong emotions from time to time. If you feel distressed by the intensity of your feelings, remember that emotions come and go.

Learn ways to manage your feelings. But be patient, change takes time.

It can be frightening to be faced with a hidden disability. But when fear becomes anxiety and/or panic, learn to interrupt the cycle and relax your mind.

Remember that most of the things that you fear will likely never occur.

Worry won't prevent misfortunes from happening.

Realize that your hidden disability may be making you stronger and more resilient in ways that you aren't even aware of yet.

CHAPTER 4

Love and Sex

*Joe and I were a typical yuppie couple. We both had good jobs and
spent our vacations at the beach or in the snow. We lived well; we had
a lot of nice things, like cars, furniture, and clothes. A couple of years
ago, I was in a car accident and fractured one of my vertebra. Even
after it supposedly healed, I still had pain. The pain has gotten worse
over the years, and I can only work part-time. Joe was supportive at
first, but he grew to resent my always having to stay home and rest.
Maybe I should have encouraged him to go out with his friends, but
I was needy and scared. One day we had a huge fight and he accused
me of being "mental." He said that I was just inventing this whole pain
syndrome to get his sympathy and attention. I was furious and stormed
out of the house. When I got back, he had packed a suitcase and left.
He's living with a friend now and going out and doing the things
we used to do. We just got into counseling to see if we can get back
together, but I'm not optimistic about it.*

—Deborah, age thirty-nine

Deborah's story is not unique. Many relationships do not survive the strain of a
hidden disability. While the divorce rate for the general population hovers

around 50 percent, the rate increases to about 75 percent when one spouse is chronically ill or in pain (Pitzele 1986).

No statistics measure the divorce rate when the spouse's disability is hidden, but it seems logical that there may be even more separations and divorces. A couple can sometimes band together when an obvious disability strikes, such as blindness or paralysis. Society recognizes these disabilities as real, and support may be more readily available. Yet when a disability is hidden, the added stressors include a world that may not recognize the problem as valid.

Your partner also has to contend with skepticism from others. Relatives may take your partner aside and urge him or her to take you to a psychiatrist. Even if your partner is trying to stand by your side, it may become difficult to maintain this faith if doctors minimize or dismiss your symptoms. Of course, your partner may be another person in your world who minimizes your disability because it's invisible. If your mate trivializes your symptoms, your relationship will likely suffer. Having him or her question whether your problems are psychosomatic may impede your emotional and physical recovery.

Yet, while some marriages flounder, like Deborah and Joe's, other relationships are strengthened by adversity. Why would one relationship disintegrate while another remains strong or grows stronger? Are there ways to prevent serious relationship problems when a mate is coping with health problems? And if a relationship becomes conflictual, is there hope for reconciliation?

This chapter explores the unique stresses and strains on a relationship when you're coping with a hidden disability. We'll explain how each partner may be unwittingly contributing to problems. We'll offer suggestions on how to strengthen relationship ties.

And what if you're not in a relationship: How can you live a fulfilling life as a single person coping with health problems? What are the most common fears when you're dating? Should you discuss your disability with people you've just met? Finding answers to these questions can alleviate anxiety and build confidence.

How Your Disability Affects Your Relationship

The impact of your hidden disability may be most powerfully felt in your relationship with your partner. He or she witnesses your mood swings, fear, and anger. Your partner stands by helplessly while you feel better on Monday, only to be laid up on Friday. He or she endures your loud tirades about the medical profession and managed care. And your significant other may be frustrated if your earning power is diminished. Not only does your partner have to help out more with the household and children, but he or she may be forced to support you financially.

Chronic illness and pain are major stressors to a marriage or relationship. Health problems are a family affair. While you're ailing, your partner is contending with challenges as well. He or she worries that your pain will get worse and is anxious about whether you'll become seriously depressed. It's common for a mate to feel angry about the changes and restrictions in his or her life brought on by your health problems.

Yet, while you, as the sick person, elicit some attention, your mate's needs often get overlooked. He or she wants to share successes, yet worries that you'll feel envious. Your partner may be reluctant to tell you about his or her worries. If your mate is stressed out about bills, for instance, he or she may not want to unduly burden you.

Since you're the one who's ill, it's easy for others to overlook your partner's distress. People might ask how you're doing and neglect to inquire about him or her. Conversations with friends focus on your predicament. While your partner is a fellow sufferer, his or her plight may go unnoticed, especially if he or she is the stoic type.

Without realizing it, you've probably established your relationship based on certain unwritten rules. A health crisis unravels the very foundation of your relationship. Take Deborah and Joe, for example—a married couple who had devoted their lives to pursuing pleasure. They worked all week and played on weekends. When Deborah became disabled, there was less money. She was also depressed and afraid to exacerbate the pain by overexerting herself.

Unwittingly, she'd violated a major tenet of the relationship: to have fun and seek pleasure. She worked fewer hours and stayed home and rested on the weekends. Joe had been faced with the dilemma of either abandoning her by going out without her or staying home and resenting her.

Even a strong partnership can be toppled. Yet many relationships remain strong and even flower. While Joe and Deborah were having major marital problems, other couples become closer during a medical crisis. Why would one relationship die and another flourish?

As an example of a marriage that is beating the odds, take Marie, a forty-two-year-old nurse who developed severe migraines five years ago. She's been married to George for about twenty years. Marie averages one or two debilitating migraines a month that last for days, so she's only working per diem. She takes strong painkillers when the headaches are particularly bad, but the medicine has unpleasant side effects, such as sleepiness and gastrointestinal problems.

Surprisingly, Marie reports that her marriage is stronger than ever. She explains:

> My marriage has been a good one. Even though our lives have focused on the kids, we've tried to make time for us as a couple. We've had a regular Saturday night "date." George is an easygoing type, so he's helped me to calm down and not get too worried about things.
>
> We had a hard time a few years into the marriage because I had a couple of miscarriages. The doctors told me I'd never be able to have children. I was depressed, and George couldn't deal with my feelings. But it helped when I asked him to just let me cry on his shoulder.
>
> When I developed the migraines, I started feeling insecure. I was

getting older anyway, and I really felt unattractive. But George reassured me, and that made me feel better.

I've been to a lot of doctors who said that my migraines were due to stress. One doctor even had the nerve to attribute them to a midlife crisis. But George has never believed that my migraines were psychosomatic. He encouraged me to find a more sympathetic doctor.

I try hard to be pleasant and upbeat when I feel okay. I'll make a special meal and focus on topics that aren't related to illness. We don't have sex as spontaneously as before because George never knows if I'm up to it. So when I feel well, we make some time to be sexual with one another.

When I first got the migraines, I was so scared that I talked about them all of the time. I could see that George was getting really overwhelmed. So now I limit how much I tell him. I call my sister or my best friend to talk when things get really bad.

I really appreciate George. He's come through for me in a big way. I'm not so bothered by the little things that would irk me. We've both realized that life isn't forever. We try to appreciate things now.

Unlike Deborah and Joe, this couple has been able to adapt to the changes brought by a hidden disability. While Deborah and Joe had centered their lives on fun and pleasure, Marie and George's marriage has more depth and substance. The miscarriages they experienced early on made them realize that life is difficult at times. They've developed the maturity to see that a strong relationship requires sacrifice, flexibility, and compromise.

Why else has this relationship become stronger?

- "My marriage has been a good one." A strong marriage has a greater chance of surviving many of life's stressors. A disability not only causes problems but also exposes the vulnerabilities in a relationship. Marie and George have been working on their problems for years. The tragedy of their miscarriages early on taught them how to stand together during crises. While their children have been their main focus, they still have found time to be together and having regular "dates."

- "George is an easygoing type." It helps when one partner can coach the other through hard times. George's even-tempered personality allows him to ride the waves of stress. He also helps his wife put problems in perspective. Problems arise when both spouses become so overwhelmed with stresses that neither can see clearly. The difficulties of a hidden disability become impossible mountains to scale. Both partners feel defeated and helpless.

- "George reassured me." Many ill people feel unattractive and undesirable. The strain of fatigue and pain shows in your face, and weight changes, along with physical deconditioning, can alter your body as well. At a time when you're questioning your desirability, your partner's reassurances about your attractiveness can help.

Conversely, if your partner is critical of your appearance, you may not only feel insecure but also be angry about his or her insensitivity. Passive-aggressive comments about the need for you to "firm up" or lose some weight can feel offensive and threatening. Your partner may be experiencing some understandable loss if you've physically changed; however, airing his or her dissatisfaction may undermine your trust in your partner and the relationship itself.

- "George has never believed that my migraines were psychosomatic." If your partner dismisses your symptoms as merely psychological, this spells trouble for the relationship. George has believed that Marie's symptoms are real and has never demeaned them. In contrast, by Joe calling Deborah "mental," he demonstrates a profound distrust in his wife.

- "When I feel well, we make some time to be sexual." A disability often changes your sex life. It's hard to be spontaneous when you're in pain. Marie and George are adapting to accommodate the changes to their sex life. When Marie feels well, she and George spend time being sexual. When she doesn't feel up to it, he doesn't guilt-trip or coerce her. They appreciate the time they can be sexual together and make the most of her healthy times.

- "I limit how much I tell him." Marie tries hard to spare George unnecessary suffering, making sure not to rely solely on him for moral support. She recognizes the burden that he is carrying and goes out of her way to be loving. And she utilizes her social support system when the pain is bad rather than stoically suffering in silence.

  Overburdening a partner is a common mistake. Given that you and your mate are living in close quarters, there's ample opportunity to ventilate. The day may begin with your recounting a difficult night's sleep, continue over breakfast as you determine what you should or shouldn't eat, and resume at the end of the day as you review the day's pain level. Your partner, feeling sorry about your pain and guilty for being healthy, may endure all of this silently—until he or she can't take it anymore. Your partner may end up packing his or her bags and leaving, like Joe, or staying and making your life miserable with passive-aggressive behavior.

  It may feel impossible at times to contain all the anxiety and frustration you're experiencing. Sometimes you may just break down and cry. But it's important to try to be aware of the impact of your hidden disability on your mate. While you don't want to become the "strong-and-silent" type and repress all your emotions, you don't want to vent them constantly either. Finding a balance between sharing but not overburdening your partner is key.

- "I really appreciate George." Marie's illness has brought the couple closer together. Marie recognizes George's devotion to her. She appreciates his strengths and forgives his flaws. George respects his wife's ability to bear great physical suffering with dignity. He realizes that life is finite, and is grateful for their time together. By recognizing what's most important in life and seeing the big picture, they accept the small irritations of daily life.

Joe, on the other hand, is still intent on building his life around pleasure. He's unable to see the opportunities hidden in any life crisis. To him, Deborah's pain represents deprivation and boredom. He may be unwilling to make the sacrifices needed to live with a spouse suffering from a disability, and he doesn't see the possibilities for closeness and intimacy. Before she developed a hidden disability, Deborah was content to pursue a hedonistic lifestyle. But her health problems have forced her to reevaluate her life and her priorities. Unfortunately, Joe may not be ready to do this, and the couple may grow apart permanently.

Rating Your Relationship

A hidden disability can test a relationship. It's easy to stay together when health is good, money is plentiful, and children are well-behaved. But when misfortune strikes, you find out how strong your relationship really is. While the wedding vow says "in sickness and in health," many people cross their fingers and hope they'll each remain healthy. If a short-term, treatable illness occurs, most relationships get through it intact. But an intractable illness that's invisible and doesn't go away may make your mate rethink the "in sickness and in health" promise.

When you take a look at the strengths and weaknesses of your own relationship, does it resemble George and Marie's? Has your hidden disability, though challenging, strengthened the relationship ties? Or has it revealed the problems in your relationship and threatened its survival, like it has for Joe and Deborah? Or has your relationship been both strengthened to some extent and weakened in other areas?

Relationship Self-Test

To strengthen your relationship, you'll want to see how it's succeeding, as well as how it's faltering. Provided is a quiz to help you assess what's working and what needs improvement. Answer the following questions about your relationship since you've developed a hidden disability:

1. My mate and I maintain similar interests. *Yes   No   Sometimes*

2. I respect my partner's need for space and separate interests.
Yes   No   Sometimes

3. My partner is still involved in activities we used to do together even if I can no longer participate. *Yes   No   Sometimes*

4. I feel okay about my mate doing things without me.
   Yes   No   Sometimes

5. We rarely have big, blowout fights. *Yes   No   Sometimes*

6. When we argue, we avoid name calling, cursing, or yelling.
   Yes   No   Sometimes

7. Even though we argue, we eventually talk things through and work out problems. *Yes   No   Sometimes*

8. My partner believes that my hidden disability is real.
   Yes   No   Sometimes

9. My significant other never implies that I'm exaggerating or faking my symptoms. *Yes   No   Sometimes*

10. My partner doesn't suggest that my symptoms are all due to stress.
    Yes   No   Sometimes

11. My mate is sympathetic to my plight. *Yes   No   Sometimes*

12. My partner supports me in my recovery. *Yes   No   Sometimes*

13. My partner participates in my medical treatment.
    Yes   No   Sometimes

14. I avoid overburdening my partner with every detail about my disability. *Yes   No   Sometimes*

15. I make sure to confide in and seek support from others, not just my partner. *Yes   No   Sometimes*

16. I spend time alone and feel comfortable doing so.
    Yes   No   Sometimes

17. I believe that my partner still finds me attractive and desirable.
    Yes   No   Sometimes

18. My partner helps me out without complaining or guilt-tripping me.
    Yes   No   Sometimes

19. We've grown closer since I've developed my hidden disability.
    Yes   No   Sometimes

20. I appreciate my partner even more now. *Yes   No   Sometimes*

21. I think my partner appreciates me more. *Yes   No   Sometimes*

22. I'm generally content with my relationship. *Yes   No   Sometimes*

23. I love my partner. *Yes   No   Sometimes*

24. I'm certain that my mate loves me. *Yes   No   Sometimes*

25. I'm content with our sex life. *Yes   No   Sometimes*

Now review your answers. Are you finding yourself circling "yes" most frequently? If so, your relationship seems to be weathering the storm well. Answers which are primarily "sometimes" reveal some stress. Mostly "no" scores expose a relationship that is rocky and fragile.

Now take a closer look at your responses. Are there any patterns that emerge? Maybe you notice that your relationship is fulfilling in some ways but not in others. Or perhaps you're carrying the burden, and your partner isn't doing his or her share. You may notice some areas where you need to work harder, for instance, in giving your partner more space. Taking a close and honest look at your answers can help you to figure what's working and what's not.

If your answers are generally "yes," consider yourself fortunate. You and your mate have a solid foundation to withstand the stresses of a hidden disability. You're compatible and have shared interests. You respect each other and are sensitive to each other's needs. You're both flexible and have adapted to the necessarily changes brought on by a health problem.

If, instead, you're checking mostly "no" and "sometimes," then your relationship may be headed for trouble. Negative responses are red flags that your relationship needs work. Consider couples counseling. Problems left unresolved will fester and grow.

The Seven Most Common Relationship Traps

As we've seen, relationships can become mired in conflict when one of the partners develops a hidden disability. From the quiz, you've detected the weaknesses in your own relationship. These weaknesses are traps where you and your partner can become stuck. The trick is to become aware of these traps so you can avoid them. And if you've gotten entangled already, there are ways to escape. Even small steps toward change can have lasting impact. Learning the common traps can help restore your relationship.

As an example of a marriage that became entrapped, take Jim and Claire, a couple married for ten years when Jim developed Crohn's disease and eventually had surgery. But his chronic intestinal pain only worsened. At first, Claire was very supporting and understanding. She arranged for second opinions, attended most doctors' appointments, and willingly assumed the sole breadwinner role.

Even when Jim's depression and hair-trigger temper became extreme, Claire never complained. Because Jim was embarrassed about having stomach problems, he withdrew and stopped seeing friends and family. She didn't want to abandon him, so she stayed home with him most weekends. Claire reassured Jim that his lack of interest in sex wasn't an issue for her. Claire ignored some obvious symptoms that she was becoming increasingly more stressed out. She developed tension headaches. She isolated herself and didn't return phone calls.

When Jim's depression became so severe that he hardly got out of bed, Claire urged him to see a therapist. He angrily accused her of implying that his problems were all in his head. Claire apologized and didn't bring up the subject again.

After about a year and a half of Jim's chronic pain and disability, Claire flew into a rage one day over a minor incident. She threw some clothes into a suitcase, grabbed her purse, and left. It was a month before Jim even knew where she went, and that was only because she called to ask him for a divorce.

Jim was shocked that Claire suddenly and impulsively left. But while her flight was dramatic, the problems were building over the course of many months. Claire could no longer bear the increasing financial burdens, lack of social contacts, and loss of sex. She felt overwhelmed and burdened by being Jim's only "counselor," and hearing day and night of his misery.

Was this marriage doomed from the start? Yes and no. Given Claire's tendency to repress her needs and please others, and Jim's unwillingness to seek help, the relationship couldn't withstand all the pressures. However, if both had acted differently, the outcome could have been more positive.

Claire was valiantly trying to be stoic, but her dissatisfaction was mounting. She overlooked both the emotional and physical signs that she was overwhelmed. Her once active social life vanished, and she focused exclusively on Jim and his problems.

Claire allowed Jim to vent continually about his pain and rage. Since he felt too ashamed to see a therapist, she assumed this role—on top of being the breadwinner, caretaker, and housekeeper. Finally, a small conflict unleashed all of her pent-up frustration and resentment; she abandoned the marriage in a desperate attempt to save herself.

Jim's focus was entirely on his pain and anguish. He stopped working, seeing friends, and doing any enjoyable activity. While his pain was real, he didn't stretch himself to see what he was capable of doing. He refused to get help even though he badly needed it. In his despair, he blinded himself to how unhappy his wife had become and was stunned when she suddenly left.

Long-term relationships in and of themselves are difficult. There are ample opportunities for making mistakes and causing hurt feelings. A hidden disability can magnify existing problems and cause new ones. The following sections cover some common relationship "traps," all of which Jim and Claire succumbed to over time.

Trap One: Becoming Exclusive

While studies have shown the health benefits of social support (and the risks of isolation), Jim and Claire depended solely on each other. Jim wouldn't see a counselor, reach out to friends, or join a support group. He felt embarrassed about his intestinal pain and hid it from others. Yet, if he had shared his problems with others, he may have been pleasantly surprised by their support and sympathy. He likely would have encountered at least a few people with similar ailments. Yet his shame kept him isolated and overly dependent on his wife.

Given Jim's emotional state and disability, Claire felt reluctant to see others. She believed that a "good wife" stayed home and took care of her husband. While she tried to repress her own needs, she couldn't contain her frustration and finally exploded.

Claire was also having difficulty with people in her life. Her best friend told her that she thought Jim's symptoms seemed "weird" and she should send him to a shrink as soon as possible. Her sister kept nagging her to get out on her own. Since Claire felt conflicted between her personal needs and Jim's demands, she avoided her friends.

But there are few couples who can tolerate the roller-coaster ride of pain and illness without social support and time alone. By focusing exclusively on each other and not creating downtime, the thread of Jim and Claire's relationship ties slowly unraveled.

Trap Two: Avoiding Conflict

Claire was frustrated with Jim for not making his own doctor's appointments, for refusing to see a therapist, and for not trying to return to at least part-time work. She resented the financial responsibilities and was anxious about paying the bills on one salary. She was hurt that Jim didn't notice her frustration.

Yet Claire never expressed her feelings directly to Jim. Given her passive personality, she secretly hoped that Jim could "mind read" and notice her unhappiness. Claire was also reluctant to talk with Jim because she didn't want to compound his worries. But Jim was too preoccupied with his own significant problems to pay much attention to Claire.

Ironically, in Claire's attempt to avoid conflict she created an explosive situation. Her leaving Jim so suddenly obviously caused enormous problems for him. While Claire thought she was protecting him, in the end, avoiding conflict was counterproductive.

Trap Three: Obsessing about Your Hidden Disability

When you develop a disability, there are now three parties involved—you, your partner, and your health problem. No minor player, your hidden disability announces itself at unexpected and unwelcome times, such as when you want to make love or during a long-awaited vacation.

The danger is that the relationship can become almost solely about your illness or pain. Jim and Claire, for instance, spoke of almost nothing but Jim's disability. Other interests or thoughts were relegated to the back burner while Claire did a slow burn.

Ask yourself the following questions to see how consumed you've become with your hidden disability:

1. I talk about it with my partner every day.   *Yes   No*

2. I often begin the day with a rundown of my problems sleeping.
   Yes   No

3. I talk about my hidden disability before bed.   *Yes   No*

4. My partner knows almost as much about my daily experiences with my disability as I do.   *Yes   No*

5. My partner has complained that I talk too much about my hidden disability.   *Yes   No*

6. My mate seems very stressed out about my disability.   *Yes   No*

7. My partner seems depressed or worried about my hidden disability.
   Yes   No

8. My significant other is the main person I talk to about my disability.
   Yes   No

If you checked yes to any of the statements, consider that you may be preoccupied with your health to the detriment of your relationship. It's inevitable that you both would be anxious during certain pivotal times, such as when you're first ill, during surgery, or when setbacks occur. However, after the initial crisis abates, you should try not to overload your mate.

What can you do to lighten your partner's load? Following are a few suggestions:

- Assume as many tasks as you can regarding your health problems, for example, making doctor's appointments, calling your insurance company, or searching the Internet for new information.

- Unless medical appointments are critical, make it okay for your partner to not attend.

- Expand your social support network.

- Join a peer support group, chat with others on the Internet, and/or find a pen pal through an organization.

- If making love is difficult when you're flared up, find other ways to be together, like hugging, bathing, and giving massages.

- When you feel better, express an interest in your mate's life. Encourage him or her to talk about what's going on in his or her work, social, and family life.

- Urge your partner to see friends or go out alone. When you're up to it, leave the house and give him or her some space to be alone.

- Have an open discussion with your partner. Does he or she feel overloaded? Find out what he or she needs to feel less stressed.

Trap Four: Unrealistic Expectations

While most fairy tales (and many Hollywood movies) end with couples living "happily ever after," life isn't a fairy tale. There are many heartaches and disappointments along the way, and couples need to learn to weather the storms. If you expect too much from your mate, you'll place additional stress on your relationship.

You can also expect too much from yourself. For instance, Jim assumed that he alone could deal with his depression. He considered it a sign of failure to ask for help. Yet, given how much he was suffering, he did a great disservice to himself and Claire by not seeing a trained professional.

What were some of Jim's other unrealistic expectations?

- He expected that Claire would serve as his therapist.

- He assumed that he needed only his wife as his major support.

- He expected that Claire would take on all the added responsibilities without complaint.

- He assumed that Claire would stick with him regardless of her own unhappiness.

You, too, might harbor unrealistic expectations for yourself and your mate. Here's a worksheet to help you to develop more realistic expectations.

List any unrealistic expectations you have of yourself:

_____

_____

_____

Next, revamp these expectations to be more realistic:

_____

_____

_____

List any unrealistic expectations you have of your partner:

_____

_____

_____

Now revise these into more realistic expectations of your partner:

_____

_____

_____

Trap Five: Avoiding Your Own Issues

When you're ill, many of your personal issues will surface. If you've struggled your whole life with feelings of shame, developing a disability that is hidden and often disqualified by others will evoke shame. If you tend to have a quick temper, assume that your temper will flare up more often when you don't feel well. If you're insecure, you may worry incessantly that your partner will abandon you.

Given that you live with another person, it's easy to project your own issues onto him or her. Rather than recognize that you fear rejection, you may complain that your partner doesn't pay enough attention to you. Instead of acknowledging your helplessness, you can become furious at your spouse for not doing more to assist you. You may find yourself blaming him or her for the problems and pressure your partner to change.

Most relationships are characterized by such projections. It's common to unconsciously select spouses who remind you of a parent—and then become frustrated at them when they act just like your mother or father. When you're ill, you can feel like a helpless child again, longing for a "parent" to rescue you and make you better.

Claire was attracted to Jim because he was forceful like her father. Unlike her, he asserted himself in the world. However, when he became ill, she found his aggressiveness to be oppressive. Rather than learn to stand up to him, she remained intimidated.

Jim hated feeling vulnerable. He was raised to be stoic and not to express emotion. When he became ill, he felt like a needy child again, which enraged him. Unconsciously, he wanted his wife to "fix" the situation, and he was furious that she couldn't.

If you aren't aware of your own issues, you run the risk of misinterpreting situations and unfairly blaming your partner. You might expect him or her to rescue you from the intolerable experience of developing a disability. It's important to realize that putting that kind of responsibility on your partner creates tension and strain.

Trap Six: Ignoring Sexual Needs

It's difficult to feel sexual when you have a hidden disability. There are numerous reasons why: For one, physical discomfort isn't a turn-on. When you're in pain, sex is the last thing on your mind. Some medications can reduce sex drive. Along with physical factors, there are emotional ones. You might feel uncomfortable with your physical appearance. You worry that making love will worsen your symptoms. And anxiety and depression, feelings commonly triggered by having a hidden disability, can diminish your sex drive.

Restricting your sex life can place a major strain on your relationship—not to mention make you feel more deprived. Like Claire, your partner might be patient at first but become increasingly more frustrated and resentful. You may wind up feeling guilty for depriving him or her of pleasure and anxious about whether your partner will remain faithful. Yet, even with limitations, there are still ways to maintain intimacy. While your sex life has changed, your relationship can still remain close and sexually satisfying. Sexuality doesn't just mean having intercourse; physical touch, kissing, and hugs are also sensual pleasures. Here are some suggestions for preserving intimacy:

- Communicate. Acknowledge that having sex isn't as easy or spontaneous as it once was.

- Find other ways to be intimate during the course of the day. Hold hands, give your mate a foot massage, leave him or her a loving note.

- Be flexible. Creativity is key. If making love in a certain position hurts, experiment; be patient with yourself and your partner.

- Try pleasuring each other in other ways, such as manual or oral sex.

- If you don't feel up to having sex, offer to pleasure your partner.

- Consider masturbation, either alone or together.

- When you're feeling better, make a date to spend some time in bed together. You don't need to pressure yourself to make up for lost time by performing sexual gymnastics. Just touching and being close can replenish your relationship.

Trap Seven: When Your Symptoms Seem Doubted

If your mate questions or disqualifies your symptoms, then your relationship may be in trouble. If your symptoms stump the doctors and you have no diagnosis, it may be natural for your partner to wonder at first if your problems are indeed physical. If you receive a controversial diagnosis with no clear cause or cure, such as multiple chemical sensitivities, he or she may express some puzzlement. And if the doctors imply that you're overreacting, your partner may not know who to believe.

But, in time, it's essential for your partner to believe in you and to accept your disability. He or she must feel okay if you ask for special accommodations. If, for example, your partner discourages you from ordering a disability placard for your car because he or she is embarrassed, you'll feel ashamed and unsupported.

Your mate will also have to contend with doubting remarks and questions from the outside world. If you request a hotel room on the ground floor and are refused, your partner needs to reinforce your demands. He or she may have to defend your health problems to relatives who make insensitive comments. If you stand firmly together, you can both cope with the lack of understanding from others.

Yet, what do you do if your mate isn't supportive? First, try to understand why. Ask yourself: Does he or she need more information? Does your partner tend to minimize all illnesses—his or her own as well? If so, your mate may have some anxiety around his or her own health, and you need to try and depersonalize his or her comments. Or maybe your disability makes your mate feel out of control. If your partner believes you're exaggerating, he or she doesn't have to face feelings of powerlessness.

After you understand more, calmly communicate your concerns. Let your partner know that it's important that he or she trusts in you. Listen to your significant other's reasons for doubt and see if any seem legitimate. You may end up having a productive conversation. It might be helpful to encourage your partner to join a support group or provide him or her with some information to peruse. Request that your partner attend a doctor visit (if you have a supportive medical professional). Seek couples counseling if you're still stuck.

However, if you can't get through to your partner, learn to set limits with disparaging comments. Let your mate know that even though he or she is entitled to his or her own opinions, insensitive remarks hurt you. Ask your partner to find nonjudgmental ways to express himself or herself or to refrain from sharing negative thoughts with you. If derogatory remarks continue leaking out, you'll have to take a long and hard look at whether your partner's attitude is taking away from your physical and emotional well-being.

The second part of this trap is assuming that your partner doesn't believe you. You might misinterpret innocuous comments as critical or deprecating. Perhaps you've become highly sensitive. If your mate says that you look depressed, you may wonder if he or she feels that your pain is all in your head. If your mate exclaims, "You look good today," you may fear that he or she is implying that you're faking your symptoms.

Notice if you've become overly defensive. You can ask your partner, as well as your friends and family, whether you seem threatened by questions about your health. If you are, discover why. Do you have doubts about whether you're ill, or guilt about "causing" your health problems? If you believe in yourself, many other people in your life will follow suit. And if you accept that your disability, though hidden, is real, you'll have less of a need to prove this to others.

Here's a technique to try to counteract defensiveness: When you notice yourself becoming defensive with your mate about your symptoms, take a deep breath. Don't feel you need to respond right away. If you can, take some time out for yourself. Try to understand the reason why you're defensive. While breathing deeply, say to yourself, "I have a hidden disability. It's real. I don't have to defend myself to anyone, not even my partner."

Gender Differences

Psychologist John Gray popularized the notion that men and women are so opposite that they seem to be from different planets. Men are "Martians" who fear intimacy and strong emotions and instead focus on fixing problems. Women are "Venusians" who seek validation through relationships and become threatened when attachments are broken (Gray 1992).

These differences become even more attenuated during a health crisis. When you're ill, you revert to earlier ways of coping. While you may have a nontraditional, egalitarian relationship, chronic illness and pain can cause partners to react in more stereotypical ways. The following sections will first describe how women typically react when they become ill and then contrast this with men's typical responses. An additional section will discuss how these responses tend to play out in same-sex relationships.

When Women Develop a Hidden Disability

Even if you're an accomplished businesswoman, when you're sick, you may feel insecure and frightened. It's common for women, when needy and scared, to seek attention and reassurance. You like to be listened to and held. A strong connection with your partner makes you feel safe.

Problems arise when your partner needs space to cope with your health problems. He may retreat into what Gray calls his "cave" to help him deal with his anxiety and frustration. Yet if you assume he's being unloving, you'll feel rejected.

Women often complain that their partner has difficulty just listening and being present. Instead, he offers advice, tells you not to worry so much, or tunes you out. Fuming, you feel totally misunderstood by him and may verbally retaliate which, in turn, leads to more fighting or withdrawal.

It's possible to maintain harmony at home when you're ill. But it's not easy. The first step is to recognize that men and women react differently to most crises, including health problems. Don't assume that your partner is unsupportive or insensitive when he's merely trying to cope the best way he can. Everyone deals with problems differently. Understand that when he distances himself from you, he may actually be trying to find his way back to being close again.

If you're upset because you feel that your partner doesn't listen to you, approach him about this. Let him know that you just want him to listen and not give advice. Tell him that his loving presence is enough. Sometimes a note, which he can read and react to privately, is more effective than a request to talk.

Recognize and appreciate what he's doing right, not just where he's lacking. If he's working hard to pay the doctor bills, consider this to be a loving act. Practice forgiveness when he makes mistakes or fails you, if his intentions are good.

When Men Develop a Hidden Disability

Typically, men react differently than women when ill. As a man, even if you've worked hard to develop your sensitive side, you may be surprised by how angry and withdrawn you've become. Since men are raised to be tough and invincible, developing a hidden disability makes you feel uncharacteristically vulnerable. You're uncomfortable with strong feelings of fear and neediness. Feeling threatened, you retreat. You use distance from others as a tried-and-true means of protection.

It's also common for men to become angry, developing a shorter fuse. Anger is a typical defense mechanism for men when they feel out of control. It's one of the few emotions that society approves of for men. Anger allows you to maintain distance from your mate. You may become hypersensitive to your partner's questions about your condition and immediately assume that she's losing trust in or respect for you.

It's no wonder that couples clash when men become disabled. To cope, men can benefit from finding ways to tolerate feelings of vulnerability. Recognize that it's normal for men to feel uncomfortable with these emotions. Find ways to recognize your value even if you can't work or your life is restricted. While you've been socialized to believe that work is your major identity, remember that you are much more than a worker.

If you feel angry much of the time, find safe ways to release your feelings. Hit a pillow, yell in the shower, write in a journal, paint. If you are venting your anger on your partner, you're likely damaging your relationship. You may want to consider counseling or a support group to find additional ways to manage your anger.

Men often complain of partners becoming overly involved in health problems. While you may minimize your illness as a way of coping, your partner is vocal about her worries and anxieties. You may feel that she's taking over. Recognize that she is trying to control you to bind anxiety. You can communicate to her that you appreciate her support and concern, adding that since you're ill, you need to feel in control of your life. Give her specific suggestions of what helps and where you'd like her to back off.

Also, notice if you're doing anything to covertly solicit her help, like "forgetting" to take your medication. Perhaps you're reluctant to make health care decisions. Your mate intervenes and takes control. But if she assumes this responsibility, you resent her for being controlling and blame her if things go awry. If you consider your partner domineering, see if you're contributing to this without realizing it.

Same-Sex Relationships

There are some notable differences between straight and gay couples struggling with a hidden disability. Lesbian relationships are sometimes marked by difficulty in maintaining boundaries. When one partner becomes disabled, it might feel like both of you are ill.

Margaret, who lives with her partner, Susan, has this to say:

> Susan and I have been together for ten years and are really close. But when I developed chronic fatigue syndrome, my illness became our disease. If I even groaned, she would run into the room and ask, anxiously, "Are you okay?"

She was worried all the time. Whenever I came back from the doctor's, I needed to give her a blow-by-blow description of everything he said. Susan would get angry if I couldn't remember everything or if I forgot to ask a question.

Once when my joints were killing me and I was lying down, she actually said, "I can't stand being in this much pain." I started getting really irritable around her, and I didn't understand why. Finally I realized that her controlling me was making me feel suffocated.

We had a big argument and the next day we finally sat down to talk. She copped to being overly controlling, but she also pointed out that I was talking constantly about my illness. We agreed that I would talk less about it, and she would try to control me less. Things have been better since we talked.

Given that women are socialized to be nurturing and emotional, it's not surprising that Margaret and Susan became enmeshed. It was hard to tell where one person started and the other ended. Once they reestablished their boundaries, they could learn to function better.

Mark and Leonard, a gay male couple struggling with Leonard's diagnosis of cancer, had the opposite struggle. As Leonard tells it:

Neither Mark nor I came from parents who could express emotions openly. My father was a career military man and Mark's was a workaholic who was rarely home. Both our mothers basically suffered silently. Neither one of us learned to develop our sensitive sides.

When I got sick, I felt uncomfortable being so dependent on others, especially Mark. I fought against this for months and got a bad case of pneumonia. I had to learn to let other people take care of me.

I know this was also hard on Mark. Caretaking didn't come naturally to him. But it's amazing to see how much he's grown. I never saw him cry before I got sick. Now he's become expressive. The illness has brought out the best in him and made me really trust him.

Like Mark and Leonard, your hidden disability may be a bridge to greater intimacy and trust—or it can destroy the fabric of your relationship. If you and your partner are willing to adapt to the new circumstances, chances are that your relationship will become more secure.

Tips for Women in Same-Sex Relationships

- Be aware if you and your partner have lost your boundaries.

- Allow some space between you both to maintain separate interests, friendships, and activities.

- Try to avoid feeling guilty if you need some time just for you.

- Be aware if you're overburdening your partner with details of your hidden disability, especially if she has a tendency to take on your pain.

Recommendations for Men in Same-Sex Relationships

- Realize that being ill may be threatening to your partner. If he's not sure how to help you, be patient.

- Communicate what you need; don't expect him to know instinctively.

- Your partner may need to learn how to be a caretaker for you since there are few role models of nurturing men. Be forgiving if he's clumsy with initial attempts to help.

- Seek support from others, not just your partner.

- Know that he may sometimes need some distance and space. Don't take this as a personal rejection.

Dating

It can be intimidating to even imagine dating after developing a hidden disability. You worry about whether you'll be appealing to another person. You fret about how much to disclose and when. You fear that the other person will reject you once he or she finds out.

Given that you're feeling undesirable (not to mention sick and in pain), it's hard to put yourself out there in the "meat market." You may wonder whether the risks of rejection are worth it. Yet, if you're longing for companionship, you might decide to take the plunge.

Alexandra, age thirty-five, was apprehensive about dating. She developed fibromyalgia a few months after separating from her husband. Not only was she reeling from the divorce, but she was also confronted with the uncertainties of a chronic illness.

Alexandra had recently turned thirty-five and was feeling pressure around her biological clock. Her mother made remarks about the "clock ticking away." Her best friend extolled the pleasures of being a new mom. Alexandra had assumed that if she wasn't married by age thirty-five, she'd have a baby on her own. But now she feared that pregnancy would worsen her symptoms. She also had serious reservations about being a single mother with a chronic illness.

Alexandra missed being married and wanted to date. But she was anxious that a man would run the other way when he discovered she had fibromyalgia. She'd had good friends who couldn't handle her illness; she wondered why a potential partner would stick around when there were so many healthy women available.

Her distress led her into therapy where she explored her fears and negative thinking. She realized that, while it's true some men may not want to hook up with a woman with a hidden disability, it doesn't mean all men would be leery. She recognized that she had many attractive qualities even if she was ill.

While Alexandra was cautious at first, eventually she started dating. She decided to take some time to become friends with the men she dated before revealing her chronic illness. One man was actually relieved to hear about it; he responded by telling her that he was diabetic.

Like Alexandra, you may be uneasy about dating. Yet you may want companionship. Bolstering your self-confidence can help you get started. Here are the four most common fears about dating, with tips for shoring yourself up and maintaining self-esteem.

Fear One: Being Rejected

Most people have some fear that they'll fall for another person and then be rejected. But when you have a hidden disability, there's more to worry about. Since you appear fine, the other person assumes that you're healthy. You're concerned that when the prospective partner finds out, he or she will flee. You might also worry that he or she will be accepting at first, but that once you've become attached, at the first sign of a relapse, you'll be abandoned and rejected. It may then be hard to trust that anyone will stick by you.

Alexandra feared that she'd fall in love with a man and he'd leave her when he found out that she had fibromyalgia. Since her disability prevented her from doing many outdoors activities, she assumed that no man would be willing to make the sacrifices. This fear was causing her great distress; she was also apprehensive about taking any risk to meet people.

Here are some ideas for coping with this fear:

- Ask yourself: Did I fear rejection before developing a hidden disability? It's convenient to blame your health for this fear, but it may be the typical way you react to meeting new people.

- Recognize that everyone has imperfections—whether it's a weight problem, addictions, depression, a quick temper. Challenge the illusion that you're "damaged" and everyone else is "perfect."

- Remember that if a potential partner rejects you because of your hidden disability, he or she may not have the maturity or strength of character that you're looking for in a mate.

- Consider sharing information about yourself in small doses. Get to know the person first and see whether you think he or she is trustworthy.

Fear Two: Being Disqualified

Alexandra also feared that men would think she was "weird" when she told them about her fibromyalgia symptoms. Since her ailments were unpredictable and puzzling, she worried that a man wouldn't believe her. The prospect of a date thinking that she was "neurotic" was scaring her off.

This fear is particularly prevalent for people who have a controversial illness, such as fibromyalgia, chronic fatigue syndrome, or multiple chemical sensitivities. Also, if your problem is undiagnosed, it's easy to assume that you'll be considered a hypochondriac. If your hidden disability is a neurological or psychiatric problem, like attention deficit disorder, bipolar disorder, or depression, you may fear being seen as "crazy."

As we've discussed, there's always the risk when interfacing with others—whether loved ones or strangers—of having your hidden disability questioned. Some people you date may make insensitive comments, while others will not. One person may express curiosity and interest, while another admonishes you about your diet. It's important not to typecast all potential partners as disqualifying and tactless.

Here are some other tips for coping:

- Don't rush to tell a person you're dating about your hidden disability. Alexandra, for instance, would usually talk about one of her friends who has fibromyalgia and check out the man's reaction. She could then gauge how open-minded he is.

- Realize that some people are truly ignorant about hidden disabilities. Once you give them information, they may be more understanding and supportive.

- Try not to let disparaging comments discourage you. Everyone is different.

- If you're dating someone, and your instincts tell you that he or she wouldn't stand by you, consider breaking off the relationship before you become too attached. For instance, be wary if your date has a history of brief relationships, as this may be a sign that he or she flees during hard times.

Fear Three: Sex

We talked earlier about the challenges of maintaining a satisfying sex life when you're saddled with a hidden disability. Yet, in many long-term relationships, there's a foundation of trust and communication that helps you adapt to changes. In a new relationship, both parties expect sex to be intense, natural, and spontaneous. When you're unattached, this pressure can inhibit you from engaging in sex.

Alexandra's fibromyalgia caused recurrent pain throughout her body. When she was flared up, even light touch hurt. Understandably, she was anxious about telling a potential lover about her special needs. Even if he were willing, she wondered whether she could enjoy sex.

Alexandra needed to recognize that her sex life had changed, but her sexuality hadn't. Sexuality isn't confined to making love; experiencing other sensual pleasures and feeling like a sexual being are essential components to sexuality. It was important for Alexandra to connect with her sensual side and to develop positive feelings about her body. To do this, she had a couple of therapeutic massages by a practitioner familiar with fibromyalgia. She also touched her body and masturbated to reawaken sexual feelings.

Alexandra gradually accepted that sex would be different now that she had fibromyalgia. She decided not to jump into a sexual relationship too quickly. When she met a man whom she trusted, she was surprised and delighted by how patient he was with her special needs.

Here are some tips for coping with your fears around sex:

- Accept that sex won't be as uncomplicated as it was before. But this doesn't mean that it won't be pleasurable.

- Remember that, given the realities of AIDS and other sexually transmitted diseases, sex now requires more communication than it did decades ago. Consider your hidden disability as just another area that necessitates communication.

- Build a foundation for trust and intimacy before embarking on sex.

- Even if you don't feel desirable right now, this doesn't mean that potential partners won't find you attractive. Try to work on your self-esteem and body image to regain confidence.

- Try this exercise: Spend a few minutes in front of the mirror. While you'll probably start criticizing your body, use thought-stopping techniques to shut off this response. Then notice something that you like about yourself. Repeat this to yourself a few times, for example, "I have pretty eyes. I have pretty eyes." Again, stop any judging thoughts. First do this exercise fully clothed. Then, when you're more comfortable, do it with part or all of your clothes off.

- There's a saying in Buddhism: "You are not your body." Everyone's body grows old. Although our society remains focused on youth and beauty, this is a myopic and superficial vantage point. It's important to go deeper inside and learn to value your mind, spirit, and soul.

Fear Four: "I'll Have Nothing to Offer"

Since you've developed a hidden disability, your life has become more restricted. You may think incessantly about your health. Since your life is limited, you worry that you'll be viewed as boring and unstimulating. Alexandra, for example, used to be an active person with many interests and friends. But when she developed fibromyalgia, even walking a few blocks became painful. She lost several friends who were uncomfortable with her restrictions. She worried that a potential partner would resent her inability to do sports, camping, and other outdoor activities.

Alexandra had always been attracted to athletes and turned off by, in her words, "couch potatoes." Her ex-husband was a triathlete. But Alexandra's abilities had changed, and her choice of men might need to as well. Now that

Alexandra was unable to do sports, she realized that she needed to broaden her perspective and date different kinds of men.

Here are some tips for dealing with the fear that you have nothing to offer:

- If you talk incessantly about your hidden disability, this may present problems when you date. Find other topics to discuss. Talk about what you can do and still enjoy.

- To combat insecurity, make a list of the qualities that you can offer a potential partner.

- Try this exercise: On a piece of paper, write down all the ways you've grown since you've developed a hidden disability. You might reflect on how you've developed more patience or greater appreciation of small joys. Keep this list with you and refer to it when you start being self-critical.

Living Solo

You may, through choice or necessity, remain single. While our society touts "couplehood" as the ideal state, being single has legitimate rewards and advantages. Being single, you won't feel guilty and anxious about stressing your partner with your hidden disability. You also won't have to contend with a partner's doubts or questions.

Alexandra was in many ways content to be single. She enjoyed her freedom and felt more peaceful alone after being in a stormy marriage. Yet she felt pressure both within herself and from others to be in a relationship. She felt like a failure being single, especially since she also felt "damaged" as a result of her fibromyalgia. Her therapist helped her to examine how her inner critic was coloring her perspective on being single. Her therapist suggested that she examine more objectively the pros and cons of being single.

You, too, might be feeling that you "should" be in a relationship without fully considering what you enjoy about the single life. Here's a worksheet to help you to gain better perspective. Even if you decide that you'd rather be in a relationship, filling out the worksheet can help you appreciate more what you like about living solo.

1. What do you enjoy about being single? _____

_____

_____

2. What would you have to give up if you were in a relationship? _____

_____

_____

3. What have you enjoyed about being in past relationships? _____

_____

_____

_____

4. How can you get some of these needs met in ways other than being in a relationship? _____

_____

_____

_____

5. In what ways do you feel pressured by the outside world to be in a relationship? _____

_____

6. In what ways are you pressuring yourself? _____

_____

7. Do you have any unrealistic expectations of what a relationship would be like? _____

_____

Alexandra realized that, while she'd prefer to be married, she relished many aspects of being single. She liked doing things her way. She felt relieved to not burden another person with the demands of her hidden disability. She also noticed that she was pressuring herself to be in a relationship immediately. She expected unrealistically that a man would rescue her from loneliness and fear. Alexandra saw that by driving herself to get married, she was distracted from being happy in the present. She committed herself to learning to be content with her life in the moment.

Lastly, Alexandra recognized that part of her internal pressure was created by outside forces. Her mother, in particular, kept pushing her to find the "right man." Alexandra decided to let her mother know that her comments were upsetting.

Here are some suggestions for being fulfilled as a single person with a hidden disability:

- Realize that most people at some point in their lives are single (whether through divorce, death, or a personal preference). Be assured that you're not the only one.

- Develop a strong support system. Since you have a medical condition, you may be worried about someone taking care of you, especially if your illness is progressive. Bolster your support by joining groups or partaking in new activities.

- Recognize that, while we live in a couple-focused society, being in a relationship is just one type of lifestyle. Recognize that media images of "perfect" families are meant to evoke insecurity and an associated need to buy new products.

- Be proud of being single. Many people who are married envy your freedom and independence.

Reminders

The challenges of a hidden disability affect your partner as well as you. But you are not responsible for your partner's happiness or suffering.

Chronic illness and pain can damage a relationship, especially one that has been fragile.

There are ways to maintain a satisfying and strong relationship, but both partners must be willing to adapt, be flexible, and communicate.

Avoid overburdening your partner and further stressing your relationship; remember to turn to friends and family, not just to your partner, for support and help.

Men and women usually react differently to chronic illness, though there are no right or wrong ways to respond. Understanding gender differences can help you to negotiate the issues raised in your relationship by your hidden disability.

If you're single, know that it's common to fear rejection while dating new people. It's okay to share information about your hidden disability slowly, at your own speed.

You can be a fulfilled single person even if you have a hidden disability.

CHAPTER 5

Parenting

*I wanted to be a completely different parent than my mother. She was
cold and unemotional. I've always put my daughter, Katie, first. I came
down with lupus when she was four. At first the doctors didn't know
what was the matter with me. I was in the hospital for a week, which
felt like an eternity. I wasn't as scared about myself as I was about
what the separation was doing to Katie. I hadn't been away from her
overnight before. Here I tried to be the perfect mother, and I felt like
I was traumatizing her anyway!*

— Ellen, age thirty-five

Arguably, the hardest yet most rewarding job in life is being a parent. Children
bring kisses, flowers, tantrums, colds, "I love you's" and "I hate you's" into your
life. One day you feel ecstatic that you created such a magical being. The next
day, when your child tells you that you're the meanest parent in the world, you
wonder why on earth you had a child.

There are innumerable books and support groups on the joys and frustrations of being a parent. Yet, curiously, next to nothing has been written about
how to do this challenging job when you're encumbered by health problems.
Being a parent is tough under the best of circumstances, especially if you shoulder the responsibility alone. But how can you endure the roller-coaster ride if
you also have a hidden disability?

A hidden disability affects not just you but everyone in your family. Children feel anxious about your health and frustrated about having less time with

you. Your spouse or partner may feel like a single parent and resent the burden. Money becomes tight. Preoccupation with your health replaces pleasurable family outings. Yet family crises and emergencies have the potential to bring people together as well as to divide them. Strong families can endure all sorts of problems and predicaments. Children can become more resourceful, compassionate, and independent.

There are ways to increase the chances that your hidden disability will bolster, not impede, your child's growth and development. The qualities that you've cultivated as a result of your illness—patience, tolerance, and wisdom—can translate into more effective parenting skills. You and your spouse have the potential to work better as a team. If you are a single parent, you can also sharpen your skills and learn new ones.

This chapter offers specific suggestions on how to fortify family ties even though you're living with a hidden disability. First, you'll see how your own experience colors your relationship with your child. Next, you'll examine your child's perception of your hidden disability according to age and developmental stage. You'll learn specific techniques to remain effective as a parent and to help your child to cope and thrive. Lastly, we'll talk about parenting effectively solo or as a couple.

Common Emotions for Parents with Hidden Disabilities

Your experience of being a parent with a hidden disability is complex and multifaceted. You may feel disappointed that you don't have the energy or capability to be physically active with your child. You envy other parents who don't have hidden disabilities. You're frustrated with your body for making it harder to be patient and calm. You may resent the burden of parenting while you're challenged by so many other problems, or feel angry when others don't recognize your hidden disability and make you feel inadequate. Along with these difficult emotions, you delight in the joys of parenting. Having a child imparts meaning to your life as you shape an impressionable little being.

Your children's reactions mirror your own. If you're highly anxious, they might be as well. If you're confident and reassuring, they'll calm down. By being aware of your experience, you'll be more sensitive to what your children are feeling. The following sections discuss typical reactions to being a parent with a hidden disability.

Guilt

Kay, a thirty-five-year-old with a six-year-old son named Brian, is a loving and capable mother. But Kay has also suffered since childhood with obsessive-compulsive disorder (OCD), which is characterized by obsessive thoughts and compulsive behavior. Although medication and psychotherapy control the more serious aspects of her problems, Kay still feels guilty that Brian is burdened with an "imperfect" mother.

Jim, a forty-five-year-old laborer, is on disability for a job-related back injury. Although devoted to his eleven-year-old son, Dylan, Jim feels guilty that he can't play sports with him anymore. He feels guilty, too, because he's verbally lashed out at Dylan when his pain has become intolerable.

One of the occupational hazards of parenthood is feeling guilty. Guilt haunts you if you work, since you fear that your child will feel neglected. You feel guilty if you don't work because you worry that your child will be dependent and overprotected. You feel guilty if you discipline, and guilty if you don't. A day out with a friend or a weekend away without your child can produce massive amounts of guilt.

When you're stricken with a hidden disability, your guilt barometer can rise off the charts. Along with the regular guilt that every parent feels, you feel guilty about having special needs when children are supposed to be central. You regret having to ask your child to turn down the television, or cancel a promised activity.

Like Kay and Jim, you might condemn yourself for bad moods or physical limitations. Even if you're doing the best you can, you punish yourself for the imaginary crime of not being the perfect parent. It's important to remember, however, that guilt adds nothing to your life except stress and discouragement.

Guilt may also cause you to react to your child in unhelpful ways. For instance, Kay overindulged Brian and bought him too many gifts. She was also too permissive with him around misbehavior. Kay needed to remind herself that she was a good mother in many ways. Her OCD was a challenge that she and Brian had to contend with, but there was no evidence that Brian was being significantly damaged. Ironically, it was only her spoiling of Brian that might hurt him.

If you feel guilty about having a hidden disability, try to diminish the thoughts that generate guilt. Guilt is unhealthy for you and your child. Like Kay, you may overindulge your child and become too lenient, though what your child really needs are structure and firm but fair discipline. Feeling guilty also distances you from your child as you remain self-focused. Following are some ways to help alleviate guilt:

- Recognize that all parents feel guilty at times.

- Find ways to manage guilt so it won't adversely affect your parenting. Remind yourself that it's not your fault that you have a hidden disability. Remember: You're doing the best you can given the circumstances.

- Children are resilient and resourceful. They can grow up strong and healthy in conditions far worse than living with a parent with a hidden disability.

- Remember that not all of your child's upsets and misbehavior have to do with your hidden disability.

- If you notice behavior in your child that concerns or distresses you, consult your pediatrician or a child therapist. Remember that seeking professional help is not a sign of failure on your part, but rather it's a sign of your love for your child.

- Forgive yourself for making mistakes. There's no blueprint for the formidable job of being a parent. Learn from your mistakes and move on.

- Connect with other parents, especially those with hidden disabilities. You'll learn that your feelings are common.

- Confront irrational and negative thoughts so they don't get you down. If you think, "I should never have been a parent. It's not fair to my children that I have a health problem," immediately stop the thoughts. Remind yourself, "I'm a good parent and my son is a good child. I can't expect myself to be perfect, and no child is perfect. I can only do the best I can."

Anxiety

Kay worries that Brian will inherit her psychiatric problems. She's anxious that her compulsive habits, such as excessive tidiness and constant checking, will cause Brian to develop OCD as well. Jim fears that his son won't love him as much since he's disabled and can't do sports. He frets that his son will develop a hair-trigger temper just like he has.

Like Kay and Jim, you might feel anxious about being a good enough parent. You fear that your mistakes will turn your child into an emotional wreck. You imagine your child spending twenty years on the psychiatrist's couch. Of course, your son or daughter is an expert in pushing your insecurity buttons with announcements like, "I'm not going to be mean to my kids when I grow up."

When you're a parent with a hidden disability, you have additional fears. You worry that your illness will damage your relationship with your children, even hurt their emotional well-being. You may be hypersensitive every time your child becomes ill, fearing they'll also develop a health problem. You worry about money. Your mind can generate an endless number of fears.

As with guilt, all parents fret about their children to some extent. Yet there's no way to predict how your children will fare. Some kids who flounder have charmed lives; others excel under difficult circumstances. As a parent, you do your best and try to have faith in your child's fortitude and resourcefulness.

If you worry excessively, try to alleviate your anxiety. Excessive worry is negative for a number of reasons. It stresses your body and mind. It's distracting and makes you a less effective parent. It's common to worry so much about your children that you overprotect them. This sends a harmful message to your child that the world is a dangerous place. Anxiety also can be alienating: Your kids may avoid you if you're overbearing or perpetually worrying.

Worried parents often produce worried children. Because anxious children fear the world, they restrict their activities. Therefore, by controlling your anxiety, your children can learn to control their own feelings of fear and anxiety. Following are some tips on how to manage your anxiety:

- Know that your children love you even if you have a hidden disability. This doesn't change how they feel about you.

- Be aware of becoming overprotective. Your fears can impede your child's development. Your child needs to learn and grow through mistakes as well as successes.

- Being a parent is an exercise in letting go. You can't control your child's destiny. You can only do the best you can.

- Adjust your expectations. You have to integrate your hidden disability into your family life. If you can't play softball together anymore, find some new activity to do together.

- There's no evidence that a health problem per se will damage children. However, how you react can be counterproductive (e.g., being too permissive or too strict).

- Seek support and validation from others. Support groups, parenting books, and chats on the Internet can be rewarding.

Anger and Frustration

Because she has OCD, Kay has difficulty tolerating messes and spills in her house. While therapy and medication help, she still has yelled at Brain for tracking in mud or spilling orange juice. Jim has lost his patience with Dylan during flare-ups. Once, when Dylan asked for expensive sneakers, Jim shouted, "Do you think I'm made of money? For God's sake, I'm not working now! Don't be so selfish!"

Your hidden disability can make you an irritable parent. You're frustrated that you can't do what you used to do, annoyed at your kids for being demanding or noisy, and indignant that you're sick yet another day. Your temper flares, and you chastise your children. The inevitable feelings of guilt and shame make you wonder whether you're a lousy parent.

How can you cope with your low frustration tolerance and not take it out on your children? Jim did a few things to tackle his problem. First, he went to his doctor and asked whether his medications could be worsening his temper. He discovered that one of his pain medications could precipitate mood swings, so he switched to another medication. Then he went to see a psychotherapist experienced in chronic pain and anger management. The therapist helped Jim gain control over his temper through techniques such as counting to ten, taking deep breaths, leaving the room for a few minutes, and repeating calming words.

Kay sat down with her son and explained in simple language that she has a problem that makes her more sensitive than other people to dirt and sloppiness. She told him that it was normal for children to be messy sometimes, and that she would try to be more tolerant. Kay also focused in therapy on ways to better manage her obsession with cleanliness, such as taking a "time-out" before responding to Brian.

Like Jim and Kay, you can find ways to control your anger so it doesn't drive a wedge in your relationship with your children. Here are some suggestions:

- Recognize that all parents get angry with their children at times; there's no such thing as a perfect, saint-like parent. However, if your anger is getting out of control, seek professional help, especially if you feel at risk of abusive behavior. Organizations like Parents United or Parental Stress have hot lines and support groups.

- Be honest with your children; explain to them that your health problems make you grumpy at times.

- Encourage your children to express their feelings. Let them know it's okay to say, "I don't think it was fair of you to yell at me." While you may not always like what your children say, it's healthy for them to release their feelings in appropriate ways.

- Apologize if you've been unfair or overreacted. Children appreciate apologies. Also, your apology can help them to learn that it's okay to say, "I'm sorry," when they make mistakes.

- Try not to personalize everything your children say or do. Their sadness may have more to do with a friend's rejection or a problem at school than it does with your hidden disability.

- Spend time by yourself or with friends. If possible, see if you can get a baby-sitter once in a while and do something relaxing. Even an hour alone can make a difference.

- If your life is overwhelming and out of control, there's more of a chance you'll be snapping at your children. See if there are responsibilities that you can eliminate or delegate.

- Make sure that the medication you're taking isn't causing mood swings, irritability, or depression. If so, work with your doctor to find a substitute.

Joy

Jim's son, Dylan, showed his father an essay he wrote for school entitled, "My Dad." It read, "My dad is always there for me. His back hurts a lot but he still helps me with my homework. He goes to my baseball games when he can. He says, 'I'm proud of you,' when I get good grades." Jim was extremely touched to read the essay. Kay's son, Brian, came home from school with some flowers he picked for his mom. He handed them to her with a big smile and said, "I love you." Kay was delighted.

Having a child can bring more joy and fulfillment than any other experience. Children are funny, affectionate, cute, and imaginative. When you're ill or in pain, their spontaneity can amaze you, and their humor make you laugh. Their charm is a welcome relief from the pain and self-focus of a hidden disability.

Although you are struggling with a hidden disability, there are moments of pleasure to savor. The trick is to focus on the times of intimacy and downplay the strains. While your children are sometimes difficult and demanding, they're also loving and generous. Focusing on their accomplishments and strengths makes you feel like a more successful parent. Here are some other ways to maximize the joy of being a parent:

- Rather than focus on what you can't do with your child, appreciate what you can do together. Children value moments of closeness more than presents and big outings. Cuddle more, give and receive back rubs, read books together, watch videos, brush your child's hair, hold hands, and hug.

- Children blossom when they receive liberal amounts of attention. Ask them questions about their lives and listen intently to their answers. Find out what they think and feel. Don't criticize or ridicule their thoughts, as naive as they may sound. Help your children to believe in themselves and to develop their own opinions.

- Praise your children when they do something right. Notice when they make an effort, even if they fail. Help them feel attractive and positive about their bodies regardless of flaws or imperfections.

- Let your children know that even though you're sometimes irritable when you're in pain, you always love them. Remind them that your health problem isn't their fault.

Your Child's Experience

Children have their own perceptions of your hidden disability due to their developmental stage, temperament, and life experiences outside the home. One child suffers from the experience of having a sick parent while another grows in empathy. While you can't always predict or control your children's reactions, you can understand their needs. The following sections discuss how children at different stages generally perceive your hidden disability.

Babies

Along with food, shelter, and love, babies need security. Their major developmental task is to learn to trust the world. Parents who provide structure and copious amounts of love generally produce happy and secure babies. Yet how is a baby's development affected if a parent has a hidden disability? If you're in bed for long periods of time, will your baby be harmed? Will he or she become more bonded to the "healthy" parent or caregiver?

Cindy, a forty-one-year-old single parent with a herniated disc, feared that her baby, Anna, would be harmed by her chronic pain condition. She couldn't pick the baby up, so she worried that bonding would be impeded. Cindy was anxious that Anna would become more attached to Cindy's mother, Helen, who helped out each day.

Cindy became hypersensitive to any perceived rejection by the baby. If Anna cried or spit up food, she assumed that the baby was rejecting her. Helen pointed out that Cindy's incessant worrying was hurting their relationship more than her back problem. Together they brainstormed ways that Cindy could facilitate bonding, for instance, having Helen place the baby on Cindy's lap.

Like Cindy, you might fear that your baby won't bond to you. Find ways to still be intimate even if you have physical limitations. Take naps with your baby, read to him or her, and cuddle. If you need to be hospitalized, try to have your baby visit, speak to him or her over the phone, and record yourself on a video or audio tape. When you return, expect some initial regression and anxiety as your baby becomes secure again in your presence. Yet remember that babies are resilient.

Toddlers

To the toddler, the whole world is magical and exciting. Once your baby can stand and walk, he or she wants to grab, hold, touch, and taste. While toddlers are delightful and fun, most parents know the challenges of the "terrible twos," where "no" becomes their favorite word and frustrations explode into full-blown temper tantrums.

When you're coping with a hidden disability, your toddler can exhaust you both physically and emotionally. Toddlers are physically larger and harder to carry, and they need physical containment during tantrums. While all parents feel overwhelmed and helpless at times with their toddler, it's easy to blame your difficulty controlling him or her on your health problems. Try not to personalize your toddler's behavior. Biting, kicking, and having tantrums are all typical for this age. Chances are your toddler would present you with some of these problems even if you didn't have a hidden disability.

Samantha, a twenty-eight-year-old mother with fibromyalgia, was out shopping with her two-year-old, Jacob, when he had a meltdown. Jacob was sitting in his stroller and demanding to be picked up. Her neck and shoulders were hurting, and she couldn't lift him. Jacob began screaming at the top of his lungs, "Pick up, pick up," while kicking his feet and trying to hit Samantha.

Another shopper, trying to be helpful, suggested that Samantha pick up Jacob. Since Samantha didn't want to explain her situation, she just politely smiled and walked away, but inside she felt like the world's worst mother. Feeling disheartened, Samantha called a friend and told her that Jacob was going to be "totally screwed up" because she couldn't always hold him. Her friend reminded her that she was a terrific mother and that toddlers frequently have tantrums in stores.

Like Samantha, you need to reassure yourself that even though you have a hidden disability, you're still a good parent. Others may not always understand your special needs, and their "helpful" advice might have the opposite effect intended. Take their comments with a grain of salt.

Some other tips: Since your physical problems may make it hard to pick up your child, see if others can assist. Having a friend go shopping with you helps if your child has tantrums. Join with other parents in support groups so that you can hear that everyone struggles, not just you.

Preschoolers

Preschoolers tend to have fewer extreme tantrums than toddlers, but they can also be demanding. Preschoolers are strong, so if they have a tantrum they can really hurt themselves or even you, especially when you have a medical condition. Holding a preschooler having a tantrum can strain your body.

This stage marks the emergence of "magical thinking," which lasts until around age eight. Children feel omnipotent, as though their thoughts control others' actions. Children need a lot of reassurance that they are not to blame for flare-ups or hospitalizations. They need to know that they can't cause your health problems or make them disappear.

For instance, four-year-old Amy was angry at her mother, who has rheumatoid arthritis, for refusing to make her pancakes. Amy bellowed, "You're a mean mother." Later, the child overheard Tanya tell a friend that her pain "was worse than ever." When Tanya noticed Amy appearing sullen and tearful, she asked her what was wrong. Amy cried, "I made you get sick." Tanya reassured her that she wasn't responsible. She also made a mental note to tell Amy in advance when she wasn't feeling well to try to prevent Amy from blaming herself.

Children at this age have a rich fantasy life, believing in ghosts and monsters and dragons. You'll want to make sure that your child doesn't have misperceptions about the cause of your hidden disability. They may believe that ghosts in the house have caused it and that getting rid of the monsters will eliminate your symptoms. They'll need age-appropriate explanations.

School-Age Children

When children enter school, their emotional and intellectual abilities burgeon. They learn social skills, build friendships, and ask more penetrating questions. The family is of primary importance, but the world has expanded to include school, peers, and outside activities.

Since school-age children have the intellectual capacity to understand more about your health problems, they may worry excessively about you. They know when you're flared up and may feel overly responsible for helping you. It's common for children to submerge their own needs out of fear of overburdening you. Unfortunately, if this tendency is left unchecked, later in life they may have difficulty expressing their needs and wishes.

For instance, eleven-year-old Marissa wanted new school clothes for the fall but felt selfish asking her mother, Carol, a single parent with diabetes. When Marissa came home from the first day of school, she was in tears, feeling embarrassed about not having stylish clothes. Carol responded to her daughter with sensitivity: "Marissa, I'm really glad you told me what's bothering you. I'm sorry that I forgot to take you shopping. Even if I'm sick sometimes, your needs are still really important to me. If something is on your mind, I want you to tell me—no matter what!"

If your children, like Marissa, put their needs second, they may become depressed or passive. They may even select friends and partners who dominate or mistreat them. Teaching your children to ask for what they need reinforces their personal value and importance.

Another potential problem for a child at this age is becoming "parentified," meaning, acting more like a little parent than a kid. This child bosses around younger siblings, monitors your medication, and insists on being the one to help you. While you may appreciate the help, this kind of behavior can cause a child to miss out on his or her childhood.

Make sure that you're not unwittingly "parentifying" your children by confiding your fears to them. While you'll want to answer your children's questions openly and honestly, too much information overwhelms them. Also, be careful not to give school-age children an excessive amount of chores and responsibilities, even if they seem willing and capable. At this age, their most important job in the world is being a kid, and too much responsibility can prevent them from focusing on this. Since you have a hidden disability, however, your children may need to help out more than other kids their age, and your child can actually benefit from being able to help you and be responsible. However, don't overdo it. Achieve a balance so that he or she isn't overly burdened.

Conversely, you may ask too little of your child. Feelings of inadequacy may compel you to do it all yourself. The result? More flare-ups and increased pain—not to mention children who don't learn self-sufficiency. Know that it's appropriate for children to help you out with tasks such as cleaning, bringing in groceries (and putting them away), and helping prepare meals. Even small children can help set the table or fold the laundry.

Along with helping your child cope at home, kids this age need to learn how to respond to questions and comments from others about your hidden disability. It's hard enough for you as an adult to field questions; your ten-year-old may be truly at a loss. Children can be cruel at times to each other, and your child may have to deal with insensitive remarks. Helping them know how to respond may empower them.

Take the example of Dakota, a nine-year-old girl whose mother, Audrey, has chronic fatigue syndrome. At school, a girl came up to Dakota and said, "My mom told me that your mom has some weird disease. She doesn't want me to play with you." Dakota came home in tears.

While furious, Audrey struggled to be calm. She explained to Dakota that some people don't understand about chronic fatigue syndrome, but that it was not a "weird" disease. She taught Dakota how to stand up for herself by saying, "My mom does not have a weird disease. She has an illness called chronic fatigue syndrome. It's not something that people catch. But if you don't want to play with me, then you don't have to." Audrey also made a mental note to locate the parent and communicate her concern.

Like Dakota, your child may confront insensitive comments from others about your hidden disability. Peers may pose intrusive questions, cast doubt on the existence of your condition, or outright reject your child. Even adults can make insensitive remarks. Children need to feel equipped to handle others' reactions. Here are some suggestions for helping your child cope:

- Ask your children about any confusing or hostile questions they've faced. Role play a scenario and help them learn to respond assertively.

- If a particular child makes an insensitive remark, consider having him or her over to your house. Then you can talk to the child about your health condition. Consider speaking with the child's parents and demystifying your hidden disability.

- Call your child's teacher and discuss how to deal with awkward situations.

- Offer to come into the class to talk to the kids about hidden health problems. Perhaps the teacher would like to initiate a health education series.

- While you want to affirm your children's feelings, it's also helpful to teach them how to ignore ignorant responses. Help them learn how to choose their battles.

- Notice how you deal with comments from others. Remember that your child may emulate you.

Teenagers

Teens turn their focus from the family to peers. These are the years of closed bedroom doors and whispered conversations with friends. It's natural and healthy for teens to affiliate more with friends than family as a way of separating and forming their own identity. They also express their need for independence by testing limits or dramatically displaying emotions. Provocative declarations like, "You don't understand anything," "You're the meanest parent I know," drop like bombs into their conversations with you.

At the same time, teens have a strong need for parental approval and attention. It seems incongruous that the same teens who yell, "Get off my back!" will feel neglected if you don't ask them about their day. Teens present a maddening test: Will you still love me and pay attention to me even though I may at times be hostile or indifferent toward you?

Adolescents whose parents have a hidden disability generally feel more conflicted about asserting their independence. On the one hand, they want to separate from you; yet they fear your becoming more disabled. Given that teens experience intense emotional states and mood swings, they may explode at you with nasty comments: "I wish I didn't have a sick mother," or, "Why do I have to be the only kid whose father can't work?" Then they feel guilty and worry about exacerbating your symptoms.

Jack, a sixteen-year-old, lives with his divorced mother who has Crohn's disease. He snaps at her frequently, especially when she's flared up. When she asks him to vacuum, he shouts, "I'm sick of doing everything around here. It sucks to have a sick mother." Afterward, Jack smokes pot to numb his guilt and shame.

In family therapy, Jack discloses that he's angry about his mother's disease because she's distracted and not always available to him. His mother counters that whenever she tries to ask him about his life, he tells her to "get out of his face." The therapist explains that Jack, like many teens, expresses sadness through anger. When overwhelmed by feelings, he only knows how to get angry or numb out.

Here are some suggestions for surviving the teen years with a hidden disability:

- Recognize that the adolescent years are tumultuous and complex. Your teen is faced with huge pressures both academically and socially.

- Don't personalize your teen's acting-out behavior or obnoxious words. If your child gets angry at you for having a hidden disability, know that he or she would blame you for something else if you were well. Adolescents are forming their own individual identities in part by clashing with you, defining themselves in opposition to you and what you value.

- Try not to feel rejected if your teen spends more time outside the house than in it. While your teen may still need to help you, encourage your teen to do the activities he or she enjoys without feeling guilty.

- While teens appear not to need you, remember that they still do. They depend on you to notice if they're depressed, check on their whereabouts, and enforce limits and consequences. A few heartfelt moments with your teen can go a long way in conveying that you genuinely care.

Talking with Children about Your Hidden Disability

Talking with your children about your hidden disability can feel as nerve wracking as your first conversation about sex. You worry about whether you'll be able to answer all of their questions. You pressure yourself to say just the right thing for fear of scarring them for life. Some dilemmas you face: How much should I share with them about my hidden disability? Should I bring it up now or wait for their questions? How do I know the right time and place to discuss my health problems?

Just like the conversation about sex, there's no perfect time or place to talk about your hidden disability. And what you say is less crucial than how you say it. If you convey information in a calm and reassuring tone, your child will feel secure. You'll want to be open and honest to instill trust. The following sections provide some other guidelines to help you feel more comfortable talking to your child.

Guideline One: Start at Your Child's Developmental Level

What you say to a four-year-old will obviously differ from what you'll tell your teen. A very young child only needs some basic facts: "You know how Mommy's tummy hurts sometimes? When it really hurts I have to rest in bed for a day or two, and this usually makes me feel much better. I have medicine from the doctor, too, and this helps. Sometimes when I need rest, Grandma will come get you and take you to her house for the day. Then I'll feel better and we can play again."

Given that children's biggest fear is being abandoned, you'll want to reinforce that someone will always be there to take care of them. Older children also need reassurance but you can offer more details, depending on their curiosity and level of understanding. Remember that all children are different, and there are few hard-and-fast rules. Some children have numerous questions, and others are satisfied with a brief explanation.

As an example, here's a conversation between Wendy, a mother with chronic fatigue syndrome, and her eight-year-old daughter, Megan.

Wendy: You know how I'm exhausted sometimes and have to stay in bed? I went to see Dr. Clark and she says that I have chronic fatigue syndrome. Have you ever heard of it?

Megan: Is it like having the flu?

Wendy: Not exactly, although sometimes I feel like I have the flu. It makes people really tired and achy.

Megan: When are you going to be all better?

Wendy: I don't know for sure. Dr. Clark is giving me some medication that may help. I'm going to read as much about it as I can and try a bunch of things to help me feel better.

Megan: Can I catch it?

Wendy: It's not like the flu. You can't catch it just because I have it.

Megan: Are you going to die?

Wendy: No, you can't die from chronic fatigue syndrome.

Megan: Who's going to take me to school?

Wendy: I'll still take you when I can, and Daddy will help out. Even though I'm sick, Daddy and I will still take care of you and give you what you need.

This mother emphasized three important points: Her illness is not life threatening, she is receiving help for herself, and Megan will be taken care of even if her mom is sick.

Teens can handle more sophisticated discussions and may ask more probing and challenging questions. Consider this dialogue between Jeff, a father with ulcerative colitis, and his seventeen-year-old daughter, Ashley.

Jeff: I wanted to let you know something. You know how I'm been going to a lot of doctors' appointments lately? It turns out that I have an ulcerative colitis, which means my colon gets inflamed and really hurts.

Ashley: Ugh, that sounds gross!

Jeff: I guess it does. But I wanted to let you know that this is why I've been in so much pain.

Ashley: Is it hereditary? Will I get it?

Jeff: That's a good question, but I don't know the answer. I'll find out and get back to you. But even if it is hereditary, you won't necessarily get it.

Ashley: Will you still be able to work?

Jeff: I think so. I hope that the medication will help. If it doesn't, the doctors can also do surgery.

Ashley: Does this mean I won't be able to go to college?

Jeff: You know how much your mom and I want you to go to college. And we have some savings put away. But you should apply to state schools, too, in case we can't afford a private school.

Ashley: Can I take the car now?

Jeff: Just a minute, Ashley. I know that you want to go, but my illness is going to have a real impact on everyone in the family. I'm going to need you to do more around the house. Everyone has to pitch in, and I'm hoping you'll be willing to help out.

Jeff offered information in clear, easy-to-understand language. He volunteered to research information that he didn't know offhand. While Jeff accepted that Ashley's self-focused questions were age appropriate, he emphasized that she needs to help out more at home.

Guideline Two: Find Out What Your Child Wants to Know

There's an old joke about a young child who asks his mother, "Where did I come from?" She nervously tells him the basic facts about the birds and bees. He looks confused, so she adds some more details. When he still looks puzzled, she says in exasperation, "What is it you want to know?" He answers, "Was it New York or New Jersey?"

Like this mother, you might be trying so hard to present your children with information that you miss what they're actually asking. Listen carefully to their understanding of your hidden disability so you can clear up misperceptions. Tune in to what they really want to know. Here's an example of an effective dialogue between Rachel, a mother with multiple chemical sensitivities, and her eleven-year-old son, Hunter.

Rachel: I want to talk to you about my health. Do you know what's going on?

Hunter: No.

Rachel: It's really okay to talk about it.

Hunter: Well, I heard Grandma say to Grandpa that she thinks you should see a shrink.

Rachel: What do you think that meant?

Hunter: Well . . .

Rachel: Hunter, it's okay to tell me. I won't get mad.

Hunter: I think she meant you're crazy or something.

Rachel: Do you think I'm crazy?

Hunter: Well, no . . . I don't know.

Rachel: Okay, let me tell you then. You know that I've been to a lot of doctors, and no one has known what's the matter with me. But I finally found a doctor who told me that I have multiple chemical sensitivities. That means that I'm extremely sensitive to different chemicals, like perfume, cleaning products, cigarettes, and dry cleaning. It's a real illness. I'm not crazy. When I'm around this stuff, I feel like I can't breathe and I get dizzy.

Hunter: Is that why you don't go out much?

Rachel: Exactly. It makes me feel sicker to go into stores, so Dad has been doing a lot of the shopping.

Hunter: Will I get it?

Rachel: No, I don't think so. And, Hunter, the doctor has given me some ideas of things to do to feel better. Our family will be okay. You don't have to worry about me. But if you have any questions about this, I want you to tell me, okay?

Rachel dispelled the myths and offered helpful information. She didn't become defensive or angry when Hunter disclosed what her mother said (although she'll want to talk with her mother soon). She reassured him that their family would be okay and kept the door open for future conversations.

Guideline Three: Don't Overburden Your Child with Information

While you want to be open and honest with your child, you don't need to go into unnecessary detail, which may just alarm him or her. For instance, this conversation between nine-year-old Cody and his mother, Sue, who has diabetes, demonstrates what not to say.

Sue: Cody, I'm really, really sick. I just found out that I have diabetes.

Cody: Are you going to die?

Sue: Not now, I don't think so. Although diabetes can cause all sorts of problems, like blindness, paralysis, kidney damage, and that sort of thing.

Cody: *(becoming agitated)* Are you going to be okay?

Sue: I think so. But diabetes is an extremely serious disease. So you're going to have to be a really good boy so that Mom doesn't get any sicker.

The mother overwhelms her child with too many scary details, doesn't reassure him, and even sets him up to feel responsible if she becomes more ill. The boy is at high risk for becoming anxious and guilt-ridden. Here's a better way for Sue to present potentially frightening information:

Sue: I wanted to let you know that I've been to the doctor, and I have diabetes. This means that my body isn't producing enough of an important chemical called insulin. So I will have to take insulin every day.

Cody: Are you going to be okay?

Sue: I sure am! I'll be giving myself injections that will keep my body healthy.

Cody: Are you going to die?

Sue: You know, a lot of people have diabetes, and they do just fine. But I can see you're worried. Do you want to come with me the next time I see the doctor? I bet he can explain to you about diabetes and you'll feel better.

Cody: Okay.

This time, Sue is straightforward but doesn't overwhelm her son with worst-case scenarios or her own fears. She affirms his feelings and comes up with a novel way to reassure him—by taking him to her next doctor's appointment.

Guideline Four: Keep Discussions Ongoing

When you talk to your five-year-old about where babies come from, the conversation doesn't stop there. You'll have other talks as he or she gets older, for instance, about birth control and AIDS. As with sex, speaking with your child about your hidden disability isn't a one-time experience. You'll want to keep the door open so your child knows he or she can approach you at any time.

Some children will naturally bring up questions and concerns; others are more reticent. While you don't want to force children to talk, check in with them occasionally to see if they have any worries. Find a nonthreatening way to approach them. One idea: Link the topic to a movie or video. For instance, you can say, "The child in this movie handled his parent's divorce by talking to his best friend. How do you deal with my health problems?" Or, "The boy in the movie felt like no one understood what it's like to have his mom get sick. Do you feel like that sometimes about my disability?"

If your children don't feel comfortable talking to you, have your partner, an older sibling, a relative, or another adult spend time with them and see how they're doing. Even if they prefer to work out their feelings alone, at least they'll know that others are concerned and available to them.

Are You an Approachable Parent?

Take this test to see if you're the type of parent a child might approach about your hidden disability.

_____ I let my children know that I'm there when they want to talk.

_____ I don't get angry at my children if they tell me negative things others say about my hidden disability.

_____ I encourage and validate my children's feelings about my health problems.

_____ I avoid sounding guilty and defensive.

_____ While I encourage free expression of feelings, my children know that making hurtful comments about my hidden disability is not acceptable.

_____ I don't lecture my children about how they should feel.

_____ I set limits if my children make hurtful comments to me about my hidden disability.

_____ I teach my children how to handle others' reactions to my hidden disability.

_____ I teach my children how to handle their fears about my hidden disability.

_____ I reassure my children that our family will be okay.

_____ I don't burden my children with my own fears.

_____ I recognize that even though my children have to help out more, they still need to be kids.

_____ I don't pressure my children to talk when they don't feel like it.

Continued on next page

_____ My children know that it's acceptable to talk with others about my hidden disability if they prefer.

If you checked all of the statements, congratulate yourself on being a truly approachable parent. If not, don't berate yourself; instead, consider making some changes that may encourage your children to approach you more often.

Parenting Together/Parenting Solo

A hidden disability, like any major stressor, has the potential to bring parents together or to weaken their bond. Children can sense if there are vulnerable spots in the parenting team and then easily undermine parental authority. So if you and your partner aren't parenting effectively as a unit, your child will figure this out.

Here are some examples of ways that parents may be undermining each other. See if any fit for you and your partner.

_____ The "well" parent becomes the primary disciplinarian. He or she is then seen as the "bad guy."

_____ To assuage guilt, the "disabled" parent overindulges the children.

_____ The "well" parent begins excluding his or her partner from decision making, thus feeling and acting like a single parent.

_____ The "well" parent feels overloaded and resentful; yet, feeling guilty, he or she doesn't assert his or her own needs.

_____ The "well" parent questions whether his or her partner is exaggerating symptoms. The "well" parent disqualifies the "disabled" parent's symptoms in front of the children.

_____ The "disabled" parent relies too much on his or her partner rather than asking friends and family to pitch in.

If you checked any of the above, there's likely friction in your marriage and family life. As an example, take Laurie's family. Laurie has fibromyalgia. Her husband, Harry, works overtime while doing most of the housework and keeping an eye on their two active teenage girls. Harry feels saddled by too much responsibility. Laurie feels guilty for being a burden. While Harry takes out his frustration by being overly strict with the girls, Laurie becomes too permissive.

In one incident, Harry got angry with one daughter and cut off her allowance for a month. Laurie thought this was too harsh, but didn't feel entitled to say anything. She ended up secretly giving her daughter money. When Harry found out, he hit the roof.

This couple is on the road to some serious marital problems, and their girls are learning to become experts at manipulation. The parents need to change their parenting style so that they present a united front. Laurie also needs to manage her guilt so she doesn't undermine Harry. He, in turn, should prioritize his responsibilities and reach out for help from others.

Here are some tips on effective parenting:

- The "well" parent shouldn't be in charge of disciplining alone; both parents should decide on discipline together.

- The "well" parent should never question the "disabled" parent's health problems in front of the children. If there are doubts, discuss these privately.

- Both parents should make time to privately air concerns and complaints. Parenting is stressful. Children can pull you apart if you let them. Communicating frequently and openly is key.

- Don't allow your child to split you. If your child tries to get you to veto a decision your partner has made, direct your child back to your partner.

- If your marriage or family life is in crisis, seek family counseling.

Being an Effective Single Parent

If you're parenting alone, you may be in the fortunate position of avoiding some of the conflict common to partners. Unless you have another adult helping you, you're the boss. Yet the responsibility of parenting solo can be overwhelming if you have a hidden disability. You don't have a person available to routinely give you a break. You don't have another person to bounce ideas off of when things aren't going the way you'd like.

Take as an example Donna, a single mother with rheumatoid arthritis (RA), and her nine-year-old daughter, Taylor. Fiercely independent, Donna detests relying on anyone. But, after weeks of working overtime, attending all of Taylor's school functions, and performing household chores, she suffers a severe flare-up. Finally Donna realizes that she can't do it all. She reaches out to her friends who have been offering for months to baby-sit. Her sister volunteers to help with cooking and cleaning. With some free moments to relax, Donna's RA improves.

As a single parent, you might feel like you have to be a superman or -woman, doing it all with little assistance. While this is hard to pull off under the best of circumstances, it's impossible when you're struggling with a hidden disability. Understandably, admitting your limitations and asking for help can make you feel inadequate. Like Donna, you feel you need to prove you can cope alone. Yet asking for help doesn't mean you are helpless. In fact, reaching out for assistance is a sign of strength.

Here are some suggestions for being an effective single parent when you have a hidden disability:

- Know when to seek help. Along with relying on your social support system, join a baby-sitting cooperative or a parents group.

- Don't use your children as confidantes. While it may be convenient to confide in your children, they'll be unduly burdened.

- Single parents and their children can be quite close. Thus, your children know your vulnerable spots. If they yell, "You don't even look sick!" don't jump for the bait. Ignoring a provocative comment is often more powerful than reacting in anger.

- Know that being a single parent is tough and having a hidden disability adds another big challenge. However, try not to compound your burden by feeling guilty.

Reminders

Being a parent under the best of circumstances is difficult. Feeling anxious, guilty, and frustrated at times is normal.

Children are surprisingly resilient. They won't necessarily be "traumatized" by your hidden disability. In fact, adversity and challenges can build character and independence.

Being open with your child, answering questions, and allaying fears will help your child to cope.

Reach out to others for help. Seek support from people who are also coping with health problems.

Having a hidden disability can put a strain on your relationship with your partner. Open communication is key to parenting well as a team. Seek couple counseling if the stresses are too great to handle on your own.

If you're a single parent, you'll need to rely on family and friends to help. Don't be ashamed to reach out. This does not mean you're inadequate; in fact, reaching out is a sign of strength.

CHAPTER **6**

Interacting with Others: Friends, Family, and Strangers

During the time that I've been sick, I've lost some close friends.
But others have stood by me. You really know who you can count
on when things get rough.

—Cindy, age thirty-four,
diagnosed with multiple sclerosis

When you're sick, loving and understanding friends and family can be a great source of comfort. Friends distract you and keep you company. With family, you may feel secure knowing that they'll always be there for you.

When you develop health problems, however, relationships become more complicated. You can't just ring up a friend and go mountain climbing. Your body has changed—and so have your abilities. While you may pride yourself on being dependable, you now need to cancel appointments at the last minute when your body gives out. Although you may have been an upbeat, cheerful person, you now struggle with episodes of depression and anxiety. You may envy your friends' vigor and health and find it hard to hear about their successes and accomplishments.

Friends and family are also struggling to adjust, since your hidden disability affects them, too. Your best friend worries that you'll get worse. Your parents feel helpless and micromanage your care. Old friendships are tested. New friendships become strained.

In many ways, your loved one's experience parallels your own. Your best friend mourns the friend who was always available for adventures, the person who spent countless hours listening to his or her problems. Now your friends may be reluctant to bother you with their concerns, which seem trivial compared to yours. They protect you from envying their achievements by withholding information from you, unintentionally undermining the friendship even more.

While relationships with others have the potential to frustrate you, they can also help you cope. Having close friends to share fun times makes you feel "normal," like a part of regular life. Being with family can make you feel secure and part of a community. Your hidden disability has the potential to strengthen and not just strain your relationships. Friends may rally around you, welcoming the opportunity to help you. Your family may be inspired by your courage. You feel grateful and appreciative of those who've stood by you.

In this chapter, we'll explore what stresses relationships—and what nourishes them. We ask, "Why do some friendships deepen when a person develops a hidden disability while others end?" and, "How can you respond sensitively to insensitive remarks by your family?" Your relationships with others in the world include not only friends and family; you're impacted by strangers as well. It can be demoralizing when a stranger makes a callous comment. What are some ways of coping in the world with a hidden disability? We'll guide you in how to respond.

Common Problems in Friendships

Judy, a thirty-two-year-old with an undiagnosed immune problem, has lost several friends since becoming ill. The demise of these friendships—along with all the other losses and changes—has been distressing. As she tells it:

> Losing friends has felt like a further insult in my life. I used to have a lot of friends from all walks of life—people I hiked with, work friends, gym acquaintances. Now that I don't do sports or go to work, my circle has narrowed to three people. Sometimes I'm angry at people for abandoning me. Other times I wonder whether I drove them away.

Perhaps you can relate to Judy's story. Since becoming ill, friendships have changed or even ended, while others have become stronger. You may resent the "fair weather friends" who stopped calling long ago. Yet whether friendships succeed or not is not always a matter of luck or other people's persistence. Your friends may need guidance from you about what you need and expect.

There are ways that you can preserve relationships—or even jump start failing ones. The first step is figuring out why the friendship floundered. The following sections discuss typical problems that friendships encounter.

"We Have Nothing in Common Anymore"

For five years, you and your best friend have skied in the winter and backpacked in the summer. On Saturday nights, you've joined friends and gone dancing. Now what happens when physical constraints prevent you from dancing and skiing?

Judy lost a close friend, Karen, when Judy had to give up sports. According to Judy: "I've been really hurt by Karen. I thought we were close, but she seems shallow to me now. She stopped calling as soon as I couldn't play softball or tennis anymore."

Karen has a different point of view:

> Yes, it's been hard not having Judy to "play" with anymore. But I stopped calling because I felt like there was no room in the friendship for me. When I'd suggest getting together, even just to hang out and watch TV, Judy was always too tired. Or she'd spend the whole conversation complaining about her aches and pains. I wanted to be supportive, but I resented her never asking me about my life. After a while it just seemed easier not to call.

What happened to this friendship? Without the glue of sports to keep their relationship cohesive, it faltered. Yet there were other problems, including Judy's self-focus and Karen's passivity. Neither friend was letting the other know that she valued the friendship. Their relationship wasn't changing to accommodate the new reality of Judy's health problems. A friendship that lacks flexibility can easily unravel during hard times.

In order for Judy and Karen to remain friends, they each have to make adjustments. While Judy may need to talk to Karen about her health problems from time to time, she should try to avoid overburdening her. A friendship that's just about illness won't last. Judy needs to also show interest in Karen's life. The two should come up with some activities to do together. Even renting a video or sharing a pizza would offer them some needed intimacy and fun.

What can be learned from their struggles?

- Find new interests to share with friends. Even if you can't rollerblade, you can still watch a TV show, discuss a political issue, or read together. The key is to focus on what you can do together.

- Acknowledge with each other the changes and losses in your friendship. Remember that change doesn't necessarily spell disaster as long as you're both willing to be flexible.

- Realize that your friend may not know how to relate to you. Be clear about what you need and expect.

- When you're especially down, you need to reach out for help. But remember to call friends when you're doing better so you don't just focus on your health.

- Express interest and enthusiasm for the good things happening in your friend's life.

"My Friend Doesn't Believe in Me"

Judy can rattle off the names of several friends who questioned or doubted her hidden disability. One friend pronounced her problem as merely stress. Another refused to believe that the illness wasn't related to Judy's "karma," while another kept talking about how he thought Judy was benefiting from being ill. An acquaintance kept urging her to go dancing with her and ignore her pain. The "hiddenness" of your disability can cause a rift with certain people. You may look okay, so friends wonder whether you're exaggerating. As Judy puts it, "After a while, I didn't want to tell people that I had this immune problem. I couldn't handle their reactions. Everyone had an opinion and wasn't shy about voicing it."

It hurts when friends make insensitive comments. You don't want to have to defend yourself to those you know and trust. After all, you're having a hard enough time supporting yourself. But before assuming that the other person is uncaring or critical, consider why they may be offering unsolicited remarks. Here are some reasons why people may doubt you. Think of one particular friend at a time and check off any that apply to that person:

_____ My friend feels helpless knowing I have a hidden disability.

_____ He or she doesn't know how to relate to me anymore, never sure what to say and not to say.

_____ By believing that my problems are merely "stress," my friend doesn't have to feel as overwhelmed.

_____ Recognizing that illness or pain can strike anyone at anytime makes my friend feel uncomfortably vulnerable because it confronts him or her with his or her own mortality.

_____ My friend holds ignorant or misguided views about illness. Perhaps he or she has read too many books that attribute illness to purely emotional problems.

_____ My friend feels frustrated or angry at me for becoming ill.

_____ My friend feels sad at losing the friend I used to be. His or her comments reflect a wish for a simple solution to my problems.

_____ Perhaps I'm being overly sensitive to my friend's comments.

Can you spot any potential reasons why your friend is coming across as dogmatic or judgmental? By considering what the feelings might be beneath the remarks, you can be more understanding. Or, you may recognize yourself as being too sensitive and presuming criticism when none is meant.

What should you do if friends voice skepticism about your hidden disability?

- First and foremost, support yourself. Know that since your disability is hidden, people at times will question your symptoms. However, don't give these people the power to depress and dishearten you.

- Educate those friends who truly are ignorant about chronic illness. Explain that your illness is real even if it's hidden.

- Notice if you're being unduly defensive. Do you immediately launch into a defense of your symptoms? Do you misinterpret a friend's curiosity as his or her doubting you? Be aware of being overly sensitive, which may derive from shame and self-doubt.

- Be open with people about how their comments hurt you. Say something like, "When you suggested that my problems are due to stress, I know that you meant well. You're really worried about me. But your statement makes me feel like you're doubting me. I need you to believe in me."

- Set limits with people who continue to express doubt about your symptoms. Say, "That's not helpful to me. I'm sick even if my disability is hidden."

- If friends continue to question you, consider whether you should put the friendship on ice. Your life is difficult enough without your being on guard with friends.

"My Friend Won't Stop Being 'Helpful'"

Judy's friend, Sara, worries a great deal about her friend. Sara frequently surfs the Internet for clues to a diagnosis for Judy. Almost every day Sara calls her with some new treatment to try. While Judy appreciates Sara's concern, her constant suggestions feel oppressive. Since Judy has taken a break from going to doctors, Sara's barrage of treatment recommendations feels unsupportive. She also starts questioning herself; perhaps she should be doing more. While Judy wants to assert herself with Sara, she fears alienating one of her few remaining friends.

Most people with hidden disabilities have several "Sara's" in their lives—well-meaning, caring people who don't know when to stop making "helpful" suggestions. While occasionally the idea is worth pursuing, it's often prohibitively expensive or has risks and side effects of its own. Or perhaps you're tired of trying new supplements and vitamins and want to spend your time living your life and not searching for a cure.

Being helpful is one way your friends manage their anxiety about your being ill. It's hard for them to feel powerless and to accept that there's nothing they can do to cure you. They hope that the next acupuncturist or the newest vitamin supplement can heal you.

Yet, their attempts to help can feel overbearing. You may even get into heated discussions; you maintain that you don't want to pursue a course of treatment, while your friend insists that you not "give up." This only increases your self-doubts about the plan you've chosen to deal with your health problems. "Maybe I should try another physical therapist," you wonder anxiously. Since these arguments aren't helping your morale or your friendship, consider trying one of the following:

- Let people know what's helpful and what's not. (Since they're not mind readers, they may genuinely not know.) For instance, Judy could say, "Thanks for caring so much that you tracked that article down. I'll go ahead and file it. But I've decided to take a break from going to doctors right now. It's only stressing me out even more."

- Don't allow other people's suggestions to throw you off your chosen course. There's often no way to know when it's right or wrong to pursue some new possibility. And there are risks no matter what you do or don't do. Trust your instincts, and support your decisions.

- If your friend continues to push treatments and doctors, have an honest talk. Let your friend know the impact his or her insistence is having on you. Invite your friend to express his or her feelings of frustration, impatience, and helplessness.

- If your friend isn't willing to back off with suggestions, you may need to take a break from the friendship for a while.

"My Friend Treats Me Like I'm Helpless"

While Judy appreciates when friends are considerate of her special needs, her friend, Ellen, is overly solicitous. Ellen opens her car door, insists on carrying her bags, and frets about how she eats. While Judy realizes that Ellen is concerned and worried, Ellen's behavior makes her feel weak and helpless. She gives in to Ellen and does less for herself than she could.

From Judy's point of view, "Ellen has been a dear friend to me. But she makes me feel like a cripple. I need to be encouraged to push myself more rather than give in." Yet, Ellen has her own perspective: "Judy has a tendency to be a martyr. She never likes to ask for help. You always have to predict what she needs. Judy would rather strain her back than ask someone to help her with a package. I love Judy and don't want her to get any worse."

Both Ellen and Judy make valid points. The problem is that neither is communicating her viewpoint to the other. Instead they're making assumptions:

Judy assumes that Ellen sees her as helpless. Ellen assumes that Judy won't ask for help if she needs it so she overprotects her. These friends need to communicate to clear up miscommunications. If asking for help is indeed uncomfortable for Judy, she needs to learn how. Ellen may have a tendency to be overly protective; she needs to avoid fostering Judy's overreliance and dependency.

If you have an overprotective friend in your life, what can you do?

- Figure out why your friend is being overly solicitous. Is it his or her personality? Is your friend like this with everyone? If so, don't take his or her behavior personally.

- Ask yourself: Am I giving off vibes that I like being protected and fretted over? Try to see if you have a role in reinforcing your friend's behavior.

- Speak with your friend. Start by letting her know how much you value your friendship. Express appreciation for all that she's done for you, but also tell her, "It's important for me to do as much as I can do, whether it's opening my own car door or carrying my own backpack. But I'll make this promise to you: If I need help, I'll let you know."

- If your friend worries that you'll overdo activities and injure yourself, say, "I'm being very careful so I don't overexert myself. But for me to get better, I have to take some small risks at times. This is the only way I can figure out what my potential is. I hope that I have your support in this."

"Unresolved Problems Are Surfacing"

If you've avoided problems with friends, these difficulties may surface with the stress of your hidden disability. Judy, for instance, has been annoyed at her friend Fran for years for monopolizing conversations. Now that Judy's developed an immune problems, she's even more impatient with her friend's monologues. While in the past, Judy generally bit her tongue in frustration, now she frequently snipes at Fran. Fran feels hurt and unfairly treated.

To remedy this problem, Judy needs to be honest with Fran and let her know of her ongoing concerns. She can say, "Fran, I know that I've been testy with you recently. I'm sorry that I haven't explained why. For a while, I've felt frustrated when we're together. I feel like you talk a lot about yourself and don't ask much about me. Maybe I contribute to the problem by not speaking up enough about my life. Your friendship is important to me, and I hope that we can work this out."

Whether this relationship is salvageable will depend on Ellen's willingness to be responsive. If she's too hurt to want to work toward change, this friendship may be at a stalemate. Or Ellen may be so self-involved that she won't stop dominating conversations.

What can be learned?

- If you're in a friendship that has been riddled with problems, these may show up in full force when you are ill.

- While you've avoided speaking up before, communicating your gripes now may be unavoidable. Perhaps by airing complaints, your friendships can be strengthened.

- If the problems aren't workable, you can put your energies into other friendships.

"My Friend Is Avoiding Me"

Judy was hurt when her good friend, Alex, stopped dropping over after work like he used to. His weekly phone calls also decreased to a couple of times a month. Judy dismissed him as one of those "fair weather friends." Alex had his own explanation:

> It's true that I don't drop over like I used to. But it's not because I don't care. I just feel weird stopping by unannounced when Judy could be sick or depressed. I don't want to intrude.
>
> And I don't call as much because I don't know what to say. When I try to cheer her up, she gets annoyed at me. I don't know whether to ask about how she feels or not. I guess I've been avoiding calling her because I don't know how to relate to her anymore.

You may also feel hurt by friends who've withdrawn. You assume the person isn't devoted to you. But there may be other reasons. Your friend may feel at a loss about how to behave. He or she wants to be helpful but doesn't want to push. Your friend may fear saying something that could make you feel more depressed. And maybe he or she is nervous being around someone who is in pain or ill.

What can you do if you're in a similar situation?

- If a friend calls or visits less, don't automatically assume that he or she doesn't care. Try to figure out why your friend is limiting contact. Is he or she the kind of person who feels uncomfortable around illness? Could your friend be concerned about intruding on your life? Consider, too, that your friend may be absorbed with problems of his or her own that have nothing to do with you. Perhaps your friend simply hasn't wanted to burden you.

- Ask yourself if you're sending the message that you want to be independent. Are you unwittingly discouraging people from coming around because you feel unworthy or because you don't want others to see you in this condition?

- Once you have a better sense of what's going on, approach your friend in a nonjudgmental way. Say, "I've noticed that you're calling less. Is there anything I've done to bother you?" Let your friend know that you value the friendship.

- Be clear with each other about expectations. For instance, if you would like your friend to still drop in without calling, tell him or her. If you're less comfortable with this now, explain why. Many rifts occur because people are reading between the lines, often incorrectly.

Keeping Friendships Strong

While Judy has felt sad about losing some friends, she relishes her friendship with Jennifer. The two were good friends before, but Judy's health problems has brought them much closer. Judy has been touched by small but significant acts of kindness by Jennifer, such as her daily phone calls during flare-ups and her casseroles.

Jennifer has also gained a great deal from Judy. She's touched by Judy's courage in facing the daily challenges of living with a hidden disability. She's inspired by her increased assertiveness as she stands up for her rights and sets limits around insensitive remarks. Seeing Judy persevere in the face of relentless pain and fatigue offers her hope that she herself could cope with a health crisis.

Why has this relationship endured while others have faltered? One explanation may simply be their compatibility. But there are other reasons as well. Jennifer possesses the maturity to stay through hard times. She sees friendship as a long-term proposition where people should remain committed. Jennifer is also not afraid to face her feelings about her own inevitable physical decline. Judy avoids overly relying on Jennifer and leans on other friends as well. When Judy feels better, she's available to Jennifer for help and support.

You, too, might find that certain friendships have become fortified. As the old expression goes, you know who your true friends are when times get tough. In fact, hardship can bring people closer together. You appreciate the other person more. As you've deepened in wisdom and understanding, your friendships have matured as well. Friends admire your tenacity and grit in facing each day exhausted and in pain. You serve as a role model for coping with adverse life circumstances.

Take the time to bolster your friendships. Here are some ways:

- Express appreciation and gratitude. Don't take friends for granted.

- When you feel up to it, do something special for your friend. This can be something simple like sending him or her a card or flowers.

- Call when you feel better, and let your friend know you want to devote this phone call to what's new in your friend's life.

- Let your friend know that it's okay to tell you if he or she ever feels overwhelmed by your health problems.

• Find ways to have fun together. Laughing has a positive effect on any relationship.

Making New Friends

You meet a new neighbor, someone you've been wanting to befriend. She speaks enthusiastically about her love of the outdoors—bird watching, camping, hiking. She invites you to join her on a jaunt. What do you say? You feel conflicted: If you tell her about your hidden disability, she may be turned off. But if you say that you don't like the outdoors, she might assume that you have nothing in common. You're caught in a no-win situation.

Making new friends becomes more complicated when you have a hidden disability. You don't know how much to disclose. Even if you've become friends, you fear rejection when he or she sees you're moody and physically limited. When you were well, if a friendship didn't last, you were disappointed. Now you're devastated and feel personally rejected. Sometimes the effort doesn't seem worth it. Yet it's important to keep your support system strong. If you've lost touch with old friends, meeting people offers new social opportunities. But how do you go about it? How do you manage your fears?

Take Liz, a twenty-eight-year-old woman with lupus. She wants to meet people but is still smarting from a rejection by a new friend, Eileen. Eileen stopped returning Liz's phone calls weeks ago. At first, Liz plummeted into deep despair. Yet, in therapy, Liz honestly appraised what happened. She realized that she inundated Eileen early on about her illness. Since Eileen was sympathetic and encouraging, Liz vented her considerable anxiety and anger. Looking back, Liz could see signs that Eileen was burning out, such as Eileen's being late for their lunch dates.

Rather than retreat from new people, Liz decided on a different approach. She'd only disclose a minimum of information until they got closer. Even then, she'd be vigilant about not overburdening the other person. She'd keep an eye out for signs that her new friend was overwhelmed.

To meet new people, it helps to review what worked and didn't work in the past. You'll also want to recognize any fears that are holding you back. Rather than look at lost relationships as failures, see them as learning opportunities. Here's a worksheet:

1. What are your biggest fears about meeting new people? _____

_____

2. Have any of these fears come true? If yes, answer the following questions:

   a. What happened? _____

   _____

   b. Was there anything you could have done differently? _____

   _____

c. What can you learn from this situation? _____

_____

d. If the other person reacted negatively, why might they have had a hard time? _____

3. If your worst fear comes true and someone doesn't want to be your friend, what are your assumptions about what this means about you?

_____

_____

4. What could be some other, less personalized explanations for why someone might not have wanted to be friends? _____

_____

5. If a new person rebuffs you, what can you remind yourself of that would be supportive? _____

_____

Here are some tips for making new friends:

• Consider slowly testing the waters by starting with only a minimum of details about your hidden disability. Then you can gauge the other person's reaction.

• Know that you have the choice to reveal your health problems or not. There are no hard and fast rules about this.

• You can't predict how others will react if you talk to them about having health problems. While some people might be turned off, others will be supportive (they themselves may even have a hidden disability).

• Remember that you're not responsible for other people's reactions.

• If your new friend seems judgmental about your hidden disability, reconsider whether you want to pursue the friendship further.

• Your own reaction influences others. For instance, if you talk about your disability confidently and matter-of-factly, others may feel more comfortable.

• Don't feel obliged to reveal more than you're comfortable disclosing. Trust your instincts, and say, "Thanks for asking, but maybe we could talk more about this some other time."

• If someone doesn't want to pursue a friendship, don't assume that there's something the matter with you. Sometimes new friendships just don't pan out.

- It's important to be your own best friend and to honor your intrinsic value and worth regardless of others' reactions.

Relating Well to Your Family

Like friends, family members may doubt your symptoms, bombard you with suggestions, or criticize your choice of treatment. Yet there's one major difference. As the old adage goes, you can choose your friends but not your family. If a close friend disqualifies your pain as psychosomatic, you can assert yourself with him or her, maybe even cooling the friendship. But what if the skeptic is your mother? Or what if your father chastises you for your newest "crazy" diet? You may be hesitant to be assertive about how you feel you deserve to be treated.

Of course, being part of a family offers distinct advantages. Families will usually stick with you through the hard times. You can generally assume that your parents, for instance, won't abandon you. If you're flared up and need medication or help with child care, your sister or cousin may be around in a crunch. Even if your parents don't live nearby, they may help with material needs, such as loaning money. And if you need a place to live, family members are often more willing to take you into their homes.

Family ties can become stronger when you're stricken with a hidden disability. Your family might surprise you with their outpouring of love and assistance. Smaller quarrels and disagreements may become trivial. You may find that you, in turn, appreciate your family more and overlook minor irritations.

Yet conflicts inevitably arise. Given your long history together, relationships with family are often more emotion laden than other alliances. After years of friction with a parent, unresolved issues may escalate when a health crisis occurs. For instance, you may have battled for years with your mother, wanting her to acknowledge your individuality and autonomy. Being ill makes you feel like a dependent kid again. Or your older sister tends to be intrusive. Yet, it's hard for you to maintain boundaries when you're sick and feeling needy.

What if your parents were abusive or alcoholics? Perhaps you've needed to distance yourself from your family. Now that you have a disability, you may need their help. Yet, you may feel naturally cautious about leaning on them now. You'll have to consider whether you can handle the extra stress of being back in contact with your family. If you reluctantly have to reconnect, seek help through a therapist so that you don't feel abused again.

Building Positive Relationships with Family

Like you, each family member is grieving your hidden disability. Your parents, in particular, may be struggling with their feelings. They've launched you into adulthood, then hoped you'd be happy and healthy. To have you in precarious health makes them worried and sad. They may blame themselves for passing on "bad genes" or not protecting you more. Other relatives may be anxious about your well-being. Your sister feels hurt that you rarely visit anymore. Cousins want to help but don't know how.

If, however, your family members make ignorant comments about your hidden disability, it's hard to be understanding. If your brother ridicules your new diet, your first reaction isn't to empathize; you get angry and offended. You're anxious enough without relatives prodding, nagging, or questioning.

It helps to see your relationships objectively. While your brother irritates you, is he helpful at other times? Might he be skeptical because he worries about you? Rather than get bogged down with annoyance, try to see your relationship from all angles. Use the following worksheet to try doing this. Think of someone in your family with whom you're having difficulty and complete the following exercise for one person at a time.

Family Member's Name _____

_____ He or she questions your choice of treatment.

_____ He or she expresses doubt over whether your problem is "real."

_____ He or she is overbearing.

_____ He or she tries to make decisions for you.

_____ He or she is overly protective.

_____ He or she pushes different treatments or health care practitioners on you.

_____ He or she talks behind your back about your hidden disability.

_____ He or she doesn't listen to what you need.

_____ He or she makes you feel helpless and dependent.

_____ He or she is overly worried.

_____ He or she gets easily frustrated with you.

_____ He or she is not interested in your health problems.

_____ He or she has been avoiding you.

_____ He or she isn't very sensitive to your feelings.

_____ He or she says things that hurt you.

_____ He or she minimizes or denies your problems.

_____ He or she exaggerates your problems.

_____ Other complaints: _____

_____

Now let's look at what's *working* in your relationship with this person:

_____ He or she has stuck by you through this difficult time.

_____ You know that he or she loves you.

_____ He or she is trying his or her best to be helpful.

_____ You feel confident that he or she will always be there for you.

_____ He or she has helped you in tangible ways (for instance, lending you money, taking you to the doctor).

_____ He or she has visited or called regularly.

_____ He or she has offered some helpful suggestions.

_____ Other ways your family member has been helpful: _____

_____

By completing this worksheet, you'll get a clearer picture of the relationship. You may note that the person is often quite helpful. Yet you may still need to respond tactfully to difficult behaviors. The following sections discuss some common scenarios and offer suggestions on how to cope.

Becoming Overprotective

Your mother calls daily and anxiously asks how you're feeling. Your father constantly e-mails you about new medical treatments. Your brother tries to make decisions for you. You wonder why everyone is so controlling. The answer may be that by trying to control you, they feel less powerless. Yet this insight alone may not make the behaviors any more tolerable. What can you do?

As an example, take Christina, a twenty-nine-year-old woman with asthma whose mother became overbearing after she was recently hospitalized. Her mother was an enormous help at first; not only did she visit her daughter daily but she fed her dog, returned her phone calls, and hassled with the insurance company.

The problems started after Christina got home. Her mother called her several times a day and became frantic if she didn't call back right away. Frustrated, Christina yelled at her to "get off my back," and then felt terribly guilty afterward.

After she calmed down, Christina realized that her mother was being overprotective because she was so anxious. She talked with her mother and agreed that the asthma attack scared them both. But she added, "Mom, you were really helpful when I was in the hospital, and I appreciate it. But your anxiety is stressing me out. I need you to trust that I can take care of myself."

If others are overprotective, consider following Christina's lead. Your loved one may need reassurance that you're coping well on your own, and setting limits on overbearing behavior helps to shore up your own confidence.

Denying or Minimizing Problems

While her mother was being overbearing, Christina's father was in denial. He kept telling her that if she'd just relax, the asthma would improve or disappear completely. When she confided her fears of a reoccurrence, her father dismissed her worries as "hysterical," which infuriated her.

Christina's father's reaction is fairly typical for those men who were raised to deny their feelings. By minimizing the potential seriousness of asthma, he avoided becoming overwhelmed by his own worries. Yet Christina ended up feeling disqualified and ridiculed.

Christina chose to both educate and confront her father. She gave him informational handouts on asthma. She also sat down with him and said, "Dad, I know that you don't want me to be sick. I don't want that either. But my asthma is real. It doesn't help when you tell me it's all in my head." Unfortunately, her father continued to downplay her concerns. She decided to avoid talking with him about her asthma.

If your family member simply dismisses your problem, you're likely frustrated and hurt. Consider letting your loved one know the impact of his or her comments. If this doesn't help, you may not want to make yourself vulnerable to further put-downs. In this case, you have the choice to avoid the topic. Don't suffer in silence. Repressing your feelings and doing a slow burn won't help your emotional or physical well-being.

Being Critical of Your Decisions

While Christina's sister supported her seeing an acupuncturist, her brother, Tom, dismissed it as "hocus pocus." He also made pejorative comments about her switch to a vegetarian diet. Not only was she angry and hurt, but she started questioning her decision to try alternative medicine.

Finally, Christina sat down with him and said, "Tom, you're entitled to your opinions about my choice of treatment. But it's really important for me to stay optimistic right now. I know that you mean well, but it would be great if you ease up a bit on the cynicism."

Tom explained that he was concerned that the diet would make her sick and malnourished. And he didn't want her to waste her money on worthless treatment. Through the conversation, Christina saw that her brother was concerned about her even though he expressed it in off-putting ways.

If people in your life criticize your current treatment, consider that they, like Tom, may be anxious about you. They're expressing their fears by criticizing your choice of action. Or maybe your family member is worried because you've stopped searching for a new doctor or a different medicine. In this society, there's pressure to do something when you're ill, even if that something has considerable risks or side effects. Your mother or brother may push you to get surgery or take a new pill in hopes for a "quick fix." Let them know that expending considerable time in search for a cure is exhausting and risky. If they continue to be unsupportive, change the topic.

Tips for Interacting Well with Family

Here are some other suggestions for creating positive relationships:

- Don't automatically assume the other person is criticizing you. Remember that your loved ones are also struggling with your health problems.

- Your family may not know how to relate to you. Take charge and help them know what you need.

- One way to do this is to communicate clearly what is helpful. It's generally better to say, "I like when you do this," rather than, "Stop doing this."

- Know that it's common to feel like a child again when you're ill, especially when interacting with your family. But remember that even though you feel childlike at times, you're an adult. You have the ultimate control over your body.

- Try to set limits with remarks or behavior that's hurtful. Change the subject, use humor, or take the person aside and speak to him or her.

- If family problems continue, consider seeing a family therapist trained in dealing with the impact of chronic illness on families.

- Invite your family to an illness support group or a meeting of a local organization.

- Provide your family with educational handouts about your hidden disability.

- Send them a copy of appendix A, which offers information to loved ones.

Interacting with Strangers

Max, a thirty-year-old with multiple sclerosis, was walking down the street when an older couple turned to stare. Seeing his unstable gait, the man yelled out, "Why don't you stay home, you drunk?!"

Marilyn, a twenty-four-year-old woman with chronic back pain, returned to her car to find a police car blocking her exit. Alarmed, she thought someone had broken into her vehicle. An officer approached her and said, "We received a call that a young, healthy woman was parked in the disabled space. Can we see your ID?"

When you're living with a hidden disability, your credibility may be questioned not just by co-workers, friends, and family, but also by total strangers. You may have to confront stares, frowns, even outright verbal abuse by people upset about your requesting special help. Strangers are confused by the paradox of your not appearing disabled yet asking for preferential treatment.

Some hidden disabilities can be a source of embarrassment as well as skepticism. People like Max who have balance problems are perceived as being drunk or high on drugs. Conditions that cause facial changes, such as Sjogren's syndrome, lupus, or rosacea, may evoke stares or intrusive questions. For instance, rosacea reddens the face; it's a challenge knowing how to respond to, "Boy, you got quite a sunburn this weekend. Were you at the beach?"

Given that the world is set up for "normal" people, looking or acting differently or asking for special accommodations can elicit skepticism or even hostility. While there may be an occasional ramp set up for the wheelchair bound, most of society is not attuned to the needs of people with hidden disabilities. Yet sometimes you have to ask for help. But while most strangers expect and even enjoy assisting someone whose disability is obvious to them, they may react negatively when asked to give special treatment to someone who looks perfectly healthy.

Marilyn, the woman with back pain, has numerous stories of awkward and contentious moments with strangers. She recalls going to the post office and waiting on a long line in excruciating pain. Finally, she got up the nerve to approach the clerk, whispered that she was in great pain, and asked for immediate service. The clerk looked skeptically at this young, attractive woman, shook her head no, and turned her back to her. Marilyn left the post office in tears.

Strangers on the street and salespeople aren't the only ones who can ignore your need for help. Neighbors and acquaintances may also doubt you. Marilyn recounted that when she was recently on bed rest, the dog next door was outside barking all day and night. Marilyn called her neighbors to explain that she had back problems and needed quiet. She was stunned when the man admonished her to mind her own business. Then he said, "It's my property and my dog and if you don't like it, buy ear plugs." Afterward, she was torn between taking further action by calling the police and her considerable fear of antagonizing him.

You probably have your own stories to tell of strangers reacting with ignorance about your health problems. Given the hidden nature of your disability, occasional negative reactions may be unavoidable. There are no clear rules about how to respond. In one situation, you may choose to argue or explain. In another case, it's best to ignore the person.

It's comforting to remember those people who have been kind and accommodating. For instance, Marilyn recalls:

> I went to a new hairstylist. I told her that I had back pain. She went out of her way to be careful when she washed and cut my hair. She even gave me a pillow for my back. I know that she spent extra time with me, but she didn't charge me any more. And most importantly, she was really nice about it. She didn't seem bothered at all.

The following is a worksheet you can use to see what can be learned from a difficult experience. Ask yourself the following questions:

1. What happened? _____

2. How did it make you feel? _____

_____

3. How did you respond? _____

_____

4. What do you wish you had done instead? _____

_____

5. What positive statement(s) can you make to yourself about this incident?

_____

While reviewing your answers, ask yourself whether there was anything you could have done differently to have prevented problems. Marilyn wondered whether she came across as too strident with her neighbor. While her neighbor might still have been hostile, she realized she might win more battles with a softened stance.

Also, consider the positive experiences you've had with strangers. Record one of these below:

1. What happened? _____

_____

2. How did this make you feel? _____

_____

3. How did you respond? _____

_____

4. What lesson can you learn from this experience? _____

_____

Remembering positive experiences offers you hope. You develop a balanced perspective of living in the world with a hidden disability. Some people will balk when you ask for help; others will give their assistance willingly. You'll encounter people who share their own story of having a hidden disability. Occasionally you'll educate and enlighten another person or win a battle for special accommodations. The challenge is to not take negative reactions personally and then feel ashamed.

What are some other ways to interact more productively with strangers?

- Pick your battles. It's not worth fighting everyone about every single affront.

- When you choose to pursue a matter, remember that you'll generally get more mileage from remaining calm and courteous. Assume that the other person is ignorant rather than callous.

- Know that it's okay to ask for what you need, whether it's special seating at an event or expedited service in a store. Predict that sometimes your request may be met with skepticism or outright rejection. When this happens, try not to personalize the other person's response; instead, remember that they may be simply ignorant of your hidden disability.

- In deciding whether to launch a fight, see whether the energy required is worth it. At the same time, consider that sometimes not responding and keeping anger inside is also depleting.

- Know your rights. If you feel you're being discriminated against, contact a disability rights group or an attorney.

- Seek support from others with hidden disabilities. They can remind you that occasional negative experiences are typical.

Reminders

Understand that your relationships with friends and family may change when you develop a health problem. You become closer to some people while other relationships become strained or even end.

Find ways to acknowledge and appreciate those who have stood by you.

Keep in mind that friends and family are also grieving. They're losing the old relationship they had with you.

Remember that you're an adult, even if you feel like a child again with family members; you're in charge of your body.

Recognize that you may have to educate people about how to help you.

Know that even if friends or family are insensitive, their intentions may be good; they just don't know the right thing to say.

Don't take negative reactions from strangers personally. Assume ignorance rather than callousness.

Choose which battles to fight and let go of the others.

CHAPTER 7

Work and Finances

I was having a pretty good day, so I went to a party that my husband's colleague was putting on. The first question someone asked me was, "So, what do you do?" I didn't know what to say. Should I be honest and tell them, "I used to be a banker, but now I'm home after surgery for cancer"? That usually makes people uncomfortable. They don't know what to say next. Or, do I just say "a banker," and then have to answer all sorts of questions? I ended up spending a lot of time by myself and pressured my husband into leaving early.

—Marcy, a fifty-year-old
cancer survivor

Work forms an integral part of most people's identity. Jobs offer structure, rewards, familiarity, and daily challenges. It's a source of pride to say, "I'm a social worker," or an "accountant" or a "carpenter." You can feel like a social pariah not having a career to discuss with others.

Yet, when you develop a hidden disability, you generally can't work as hard as you did before. If you were a workaholic, you have to set limits on your compulsivity. Fatigue and pain may distract you. Your productivity may be down due to sick days. Often, you have to give up exciting opportunities, such as traveling or new projects. Perhaps you've switched from working full-time to working part-time. And what might be most difficult is having to take a temporary or permanent leave from the work world.

Society is built on the Protestant work ethic which compels citizens to work hard each day. Full-time mothers have complained for decades that they're devalued because they don't earn money. Those workers who put in sixty-hour work weeks, sacrificing personal needs and family, are rewarded by larger paychecks and corner offices. With downsizing in the 21st century and the diminished power of unions, employees live with job insecurity as well as larger workloads.

With this type of pressure, developing a hidden disability can make you feel like Sisyphus, pushing that proverbial boulder up the mountain, only to have it slide down again. You try to maintain the same frantic pace, denying your special needs. You feel conflicted about whether to keep your disability a secret and maintain your privacy, yet you need some relief and special accommodations. Feeling helpless and overloaded, you find yourself exhausted and in more pain at the end of the day.

If you've left the job force, you may feel like Marcy, unsure about how to tell others and lost without a job identity. You may be reluctant to talk about your hidden disability, fearing intrusive questions or awkward silences. Not working can make you feel inferior to others or envious of their successes or stimulating careers.

The challenges of working with a hidden disability can be daunting. Yet it's essential to find ways to manage, maintain your dignity, and take care of yourself. In this chapter, we'll teach you how to notice and combat work stress. You'll learn techniques for coping with difficult bosses and co-workers. Your rights on the job will be described. You'll also learn coping skills to use when you can't work, as well as strategies for job hunting.

Are You Stressed Out?

Work can be hazardous to your health. Even when you're well, overworking can exhaust you and make you vulnerable to viruses and flus. And when you live with a hidden disability, work stress can worsen your physical symptoms. If you think you're burning out on your job, then it's time to make significant and practical changes. See if you're engaging in any of the following potentially hazardous behaviors:

_____ working overtime

_____ taking work home (literally)

_____ taking work home (mentally)

_____ volunteering to do more than you can handle

_____ not taking rest breaks

_____ not taking your full lunch break

_____ staying inside every lunch break

_____ not stretching routinely

_____ not setting limits with co-workers who dump work on you

_____ not setting limits with co-workers who are difficult or intrusive

_____ not asking for special accommodations for your hidden disability (whether to disclose or not—is a tricky question that we'll discuss more later in this chapter)

_____ not taking vacations

_____ going to work ill

_____ getting angry at yourself for not working as hard as you used to

_____ displacing frustration from the day onto others (i.e., partner, children, friends)

_____ getting irritable with co-workers because of your pain or fatigue

_____ acting out at work, by doing things such as missing deadlines or coming in late

_____ ignoring your body's warning signs that it's overly stressed

_____ spending the weekend recuperating from the week

_____ isolating yourself from others at work

_____ other risky behavior: _____

Do any of these sound familiar? If you checked one or more, then your work habits may be jeopardizing your health. You need to figure out why you are maintaining a pace that overwhelms you. For instance, if you're a type A person, slowing down may feel torturous, so you continue at a rapid pace. Teri, a stockbroker recently diagnosed with chronic fatigue syndrome, had this to say, "I'm a type A person trapped in a type Z body, and I just want to scream!"

In addition to feeling frustrated, you probably feel sad about having to slow down. If you've focused your life on career, having to reduce your pace represents a major loss. It's also scary in our competitive, high-pressure work world to not be a workaholic. You fear being left in the dust while others achieve success. Or you fear that someday you won't be able to work at all.

There may be a few different reasons why you're maintaining a frenzied pace. You need to first figure out what's driving you before you can learn how to slow down. Here's a technique that explores your feelings about work. In the first column, write down all of your concerns about slowing down. In the next column, record your emotions. In the third column, indicate the advantages of slowing down.

Symptoms of Burnout

Given your health problems, it's risky to get burned out on work. The result may be increased pain or new symptoms. Learn to heed the symptoms of burnout. Here are a few:

- worsening of your physical symptoms
- frequently catching colds or flues
- "acting out" your work stress, for instance, being late to work, forgetting to return phone calls, not meeting deadlines
- complaining incessantly to others
- increased feelings of depression, anger, and anxiety
- losing interest in work as well as the rest of your life
- being exhausted
- use of alcohol or drugs to try to relax
- too much television watching

Below is the chart that Teri, the stockbroker with CFIDS, created:

If I start slowing down:	Emotions:
I have to acknowledge I'm ill.	sadness, loss, fear, relief
I may lose the respect of my boss and co-workers.	embarrassment, shame
I won't do as well as others.	envy, competition
I'll feel weak and inferior.	self-hate
I may lose my job.	fear, sadness, anger

Next, Teri added in the third column the advantages of slowing down.

If I start slowing down:	Emotions:	Advantages of slowing down:
I have to acknowledge I'm ill.	sadness, loss, fear, relief	I'll get some rest.
I may lose the respect of my boss and co-workers.	embarrassment, shame	I'll learn to stop worrying so much about others' opinions of me.

If I start slowing down:	Emotions:	Advantages of slowing down:
I won't do as well as others.	envy, competition	I don't know this for a fact.
I'll feel weak and inferior.	self-hate	I'll learn to love myself anyway.
I may lose my job.	fear, sadness, anger	Maybe it's better in the long run for me to do work that's less demanding.

Here's a worksheet for you to try this exercise. After you see what's producing the inner drive to overwork, you can take steps to alleviate the pressure.

If I start slowing down:	Emotions:	Advantages of slowing down:

While doing this exercise, remember that not of all your concerns about work are irrational. If your company is highly competitive and layoffs are looming, there are legitimate reasons to worry if you aren't producing like others. But ask yourself: How much do you want to work in such an environment? Are there workplaces in your field that are more supportive? Granted, you might have to take a salary cut or a demotion, but the benefits of decreased pressure may outweigh the losses of leaving your current job.

If you're the sole breadwinner in your family with little financial help from others, then you have more at stake. Also, if you're in a field with limited opportunities, you may worry with good cause about even finding another job. Each person's situation is unique, and there are no hard and fast rules. Your friends' advice to not overwork is less helpful if you are a single parent, for example. But if work is producing new symptoms or intensifying old ones, looking at alternatives is essential.

Letting Go

Relieving work stress not only means modifying your habits but also adjusting your attitude. This means letting go of your expectations of yourself as a worker—admittedly not an easy task. You probably feel anxious at the prospect of making changes at work. While you realize deep inside that you need to slow down, another part of you fights this truth. It feels that by letting go, you're relinquishing control over your life.

But letting go doesn't mean losing yourself. It actually symbolizes accepting and expanding your life. Holding on causes you further emotional suffering and increased disability. Letting go and allowing your life to unfold is a loving and compassionate act. It's also an inevitable lesson that every person must learn at some point, as all of us age, grow ill, and experience disappointments and failures. To paraphrase meditation teacher Jack Kornfeld: If you don't learn to let go during the course of your life, you get a crash course at the end.

You may hold on in part because you fear colleagues finding out about your hidden disability. You dread people's pity or judgments. Appearing "normal" seems essential to fitting in with those around you. While you fear others' disbelief or scorn, it's important to do a reality check because not everybody will respond with criticism or disbelief. Be mindful of projecting your fears onto other people and seeing ridicule or skepticism where there is none.

Acknowledge how upsetting it is to change your work life in any way. You have certain dreams and goals you've hoped to fulfill. Letting go of some of these dreams for now is a significant loss, and it's natural to feel uneasy. Perhaps at a later date you'll have more opportunities at work, perhaps not. No one can predict the future. Remind yourself as many times as you need to that your main commitment is to your health.

While you feel pride in working in a certain capacity, remember that you are valuable as a person far beyond your work life. There may be possibilities in store for your life that you can't even imagine. Persevering with pain and illness can make a person deeper and wiser. Closing one door allows another to open.

For instance, Teri, a stockbroker, learned this lesson when she needed to take a leave of absence from work. She felt despondent to have to take this respite and worried that clients and colleagues would think less of her.

After about a month at home, where she became increasingly more demoralized, Teri resolved to use her time productively. She had always loved drawing but hadn't drawn in years. Spending time each week immersed in her artwork, she rediscovered her love for drawing. After she started feeling better, she vowed to continue her art.

What Are Your Special Needs?

As a person with a hidden disability, you may have special requirements in the work place. An ergonomic chair, flexible work schedule, or diversified job duties may allow you to work more comfortably and efficiently. Yet advocating for yourself isn't so easy. Not only do you have to figure out what you need, you also have to feel entitled to ask.

Consider Joanne, a forty-eight-year-old paralegal with severe back pain, who has been trying to maintain her usual fifty-hour work week. Her job requires hours of sitting at her computer, which amplifies her pain. She feels trapped: She assumes that her demanding boss will be unsympathetic and yet she is skeptical about getting another well-paying job. While her husband works, their expenses are considerable.

Joanne realizes that her current situation is intolerable. She's irritable with her kids when she gets home. She drinks copious amounts of caffeine to get through the day and takes Vicodin at night to sleep. Her husband balks at having to do all the housework over the weekend while she recovers.

Joanne decides to see a therapist to help her become mobilized. The therapist recommends the following process: first, review her options; second, decide on a plan of action; third, identify her special needs; and fourth, advocate for those needs.

Joanne began by mapping out her options with the pros and cons of each choice:

Options	Pros	Cons
do nothing	job security	pain!
stay and say something	decreased pain	ridicule of boss
get new job	find better situation	fears of unemployment, maybe a worse boss
not work for a while	rest and recuperation	have to pull kids out of private school

Second, Joanne chose a plan. While none of her options was perfect, Joanne decided to stay for the time being and speak with her boss. Third, she listed her special accommodations that, if met, would better enable her to perform her job duties. These accommodations were: an ergonomic chair, a five-minute stretch break every hour, a full lunch hour each day where she can take a brief walk (before she'd been downing a sandwich while working), and some diversity of tasks, such as photocopying or mailing letters, which would give her a break from sitting.

In looking at her list, Joan realized it wasn't just her employer who needed to make changes; she was contributing to her pain by her relentless pace. She resolved to take short walks at lunch, do simple stretches during the day, and socialize with others.

Lastly, in therapy, Joanne tried to anticipate her boss's arguments and practiced possible responses. She and her therapist role played various scenarios. When she finally met with her supervisor, Jack, she was prepared and confident. This was how the conversation went after Joanne described her back problem and special needs:

Jack: Joanne, do you realize that someone will have to do extra work, that we'll have to increase another paralegal's workload to accommodate you?

Joanne: This certainly isn't my intention. But I do know that I need to protect my back while still doing the best work that I can.

Jack: Are you sure you want to work here? Maybe this job is just too stressful for you.

Joanne: My job is very important to me. I'm sure that once my special needs are accommodated, I will continue to be a very productive worker.

Jack: You know Marty in litigation? He hurt his back playing golf and was laid up for a few weeks. He went to this chiropractor and feels terrific. Maybe you should get his chiropractor's name.

Joanne: I appreciate your concern, Jack. But my back problem is due to a herniated disc and not an injury. I would be glad to get you a note from my doctor about the condition.

By asserting herself, Joanne knew that she was taking some risks. He could overtly reject her request, forcing her to go above his head and alienate him. Her job could be on the line. But she realized that she had to take the chance. As it turned out, after some initial skepticism, her supervisor accommodated her requests.

Like Joanne, you need to see that you have choices and options, although none may be risk-free. Here's a worksheet to map out your own unique situation. First determine the pros and cons of each option you can think of:

Options	Pros	Cons

Now weigh the pros and cons and decide on one or more of the options:

The options you've decided on are: _____

_____

Your special needs are: _____

_____

You will tell your supervisor the following about your special needs:

_____

_____

_____

Your supervisor will probably say: _____

_____

If your supervisor does say this, you can respond by: _____

_____

_____

Your supervisor might also say: _____

_____

To this, you can respond by: _____

_____

_____

Should You Disclose?

Whether or not to tell your supervisor or co-workers about your hidden disability is a major decision. While laws protect you against blatant abuse, you may have to deal with subtle discrimination. Your decision to disclose or not is a personal one, that you should make after considering the risks versus the benefits.

If your co-workers and managers are supportive and respectful, then you may be able to speak freely about your hidden disability. If you instead work in a competitive or conflictual atmosphere with untrustworthy co-workers and bosses, then you'll need to seriously consider the potential ramifications. Consider, too, your type of hidden disability. Controversial diagnoses, such as multiple chemical sensitivities, may be met with suspicion or ridicule. If you reveal a psychiatric disability, supervisors and colleagues could react with aversion or anxiety. You'll need to examine the full picture: your work environment, your hidden disability, and how pressing your need is for special accommodations.

Following are some potential pros about disclosing. Check all that apply:

_____   You'll be able to work at a more reasonable pace.

_____   You'll obtain special accommodations, such as an ergonomic chair or an improved workstation.

_____   You'll receive assistance from others, such as someone to help you photocopy materials.

_____   You'll be able to stop working overtime.

_____   Your boss will be more understanding if your productivity goes down.

_____   Your co-workers will be more understanding if your productivity goes down.

_____   You'll be able to take more rest breaks and/or your full lunch hours.

_____   You'll feel relieved to have people know.

_____   You may learn that others are also dealing with a hidden disability.

_____   You won't be hassled so much if you take sick leave or go to doctor's appointments.

_____   You'll be able to do work at home or have flexible hours.

_____   Other potential benefits: _____

_____

The risks of your disclosing are:

_____   You may get fired.

_____   You may lose your boss's respect.

_____   You may lose your co-workers' respect.

_____   Others may be skeptical, thinking you're exaggerating to get special privileges.

_____   You may lose special projects.

_____   You may lose out on your raise.

_____   You may lose out on your promotion.

_____   Others may make disparaging comments.

_____   Others may become too intrusive in your life.

_____ People may feel sorry for you.

_____ You may feel exposed and on display.

_____ You may feel alienated from others.

_____ You'll have to contend with other people's envy or resentment at your being treated as "special."

_____ You'll lose your privacy.

_____ Other potential risks: _____

_____

Taking a close look at your list can be illuminating. You may realize that there are more potential benefits than risks. Or you may see the opposite—that the risks aren't worth it at this point in time. Or perhaps you'll learn that your situation is mixed, that there are many pros as well as cons. The reality is that you cannot totally predict the reactions of others. Since workplaces are often in flux, your supportive supervisor may leave only to be replaced by someone who thinks illness is a defect of character.

Speak with people whom you trust about whether to disclose or not. Then decide based on the information you have on hand now. Remember to support yourself. If you tell others and meet with skepticism, you have nothing to feel ashamed of. Your hidden disability is real even if others doubt you. And although you have special needs, you are a valuable and worthwhile member of your workplace.

Coping with Difficult Supervisors

Perhaps you're fortunate: your supervisor is capable and proactive. She or he recognizes your special needs and advocates for you with upper managers. Or maybe your boss is like Joanne's, a taskmaster who expects long hours without complaint. If you're stuck with an unreasonable supervisor, you need strategies for survival. The following sections discuss some common examples of difficult supervisors and ways to cope with them.

The Skeptical Boss

This boss wonders whether you're malingering, claiming to be disabled to avoid certain responsibilities. He or she makes comments like, "I have migraines, but I never take sick leave."

Strategies

First, support yourself so you don't let your boss's doubt undermine your self-confidence. Remind yourself that, since your disability is hidden, people may question whether you're really disabled. Remember that you have a right to accommodations regardless of what your boss may say.

His or her boasting about not taking sick leave may make you feel inferior. Remember: It's his or her choice to work while in pain. As you've discovered, overworking while ill is not a badge of courage—it's short-sighted and risky.

When dealing with this type of supervisor, try your best to not be defensive. Avoid going into lengthy explanations of your problems. Offer to provide him or her with medical documentation. Say to your boss, "I'm glad that you're able to work with migraines. But my carpal tunnel syndrome requires me to take stretch breaks throughout the day. I'd be glad to discuss when it would be best to take these breaks."

The Passive-Aggressive Boss

This kind of boss smiles at your requests but inside seethes. He or she likes to dominate the staff and is frustrated that he or she can't control you. This boss "forgets" to respond to your requests, talks behind your back, and is late for meetings with you.

Strategies

Put everything in writing. Don't ask verbally for a special chair; write it down in a memo or e-mail (keeping copies for yourself) and request a response within a specified time frame. Follow up two weeks later with a second memo or e-mail and request a definite date for the chair. Express doubts in the memo about your ability to do your work productively without your new chair. You might want to add that you're hoping to avoid taking leave but may have to if you don't receive your chair by a certain date. If this doesn't work, you'll need to contact your human resources department or a higher level manager.

Resist the temptation to respond to his or her passive-aggressiveness in the same way or with outright hostility. Ignore passive-aggressive comments and don't personalize them. If this doesn't work, tactfully confront your boss: "I'm not sure I understand what you're saying. Are you bothered by something?"

The Passive Boss

The passive boss is affable but doesn't like making waves. While sympathetic to your plight, this boss isn't willing to advocate for you, directing you to others although only he or she has the power to help you. The passive boss promises to assist but is evasive as to how or when.

Strategies

Make this boss's job as easy as possible. Have a plan in mind before speaking with a passive boss. Then be clear about what you want. If you want to work at home, outline this plan in writing with a potential start-up date. Don't ask, "Can I start this next month?" Instead, inquire, "Would you prefer I start this October 1 or November 1?" If he's noncommittal, say, "Let's pilot this for two months starting October 1. We can then evaluate how this is working for the company."

The Hostile Boss

This supervisor ridicules you outright for needing special accommodations. He or she singles you out at meetings with remarks like, "This project has a June 1 deadline. Sarah, with your stomach problems and all, will we be able to count on you?" The hostile boss patronizes you when you take off for medical appointments. He or she gives you a smaller bonus and a negative performance review for reasons directly related to your disability.

Strategies

This supervisor's behavior borders on harassment. You need to figure out an immediate approach so you're not flattened by his or her abuse. You may need to meet with your boss and say, "I have appreciated our working relationship, so I want to be straightforward with you. I know you're frustrated by my having a disability, but I'm uncomfortable about how you're expressing it."

If your boss continues to harass you, then you'll have to choose a decisive course of action. You'll need to speak to an upper manager, a human resources professional, or a counselor from employee assistance. Consider consulting with an attorney about your legal rights. If nothing stops his or her hostility, you'll need to leave to preserve your emotional and physical well-being. Make sure to document all dates and describe these incidents in detail.

The Intrusive Supervisor

This boss frequently asks how you're feeling, touching your shoulder to let you know he or she is concerned. This supervisor brings you articles on vitamins and acupuncture and asks you about your doctor appointments.

Strategies

When the intrusive boss asks about your health, say, "Thank you for your concern." Then immediately change the subject to a work issue. If he or she doesn't take the hint, say, "I appreciate all of your support and concern. But at work I really want to focus on my responsibilities here, not my health."

What If You're Unfairly Treated?

After you've discussed your hidden disability with your boss, hopefully he or she will be responsive and respectful. Unfortunately, a small number of managers may retaliate through unfair treatment, such as negative performance reviews or even terminations.

For instance, Sandy, a forty-two-year-old project manager who had been recently hospitalized for severe depression, asked her boss to allow her to work at home ten hours per week. Her boss authorized this and even set her up with a computer at home. Sandy felt that she was as productive as ever so was shocked and distressed when she received a negative performance review. While her boss avoided any mention of her hidden disability, he downgraded her on teamwork and communication skills. The raise she anticipated was deferred.

During the review, Sandy asked whether the negative evaluation had anything to do with her recent hospitalization. Her supervisor said "no" and cited a couple of somewhat vague examples of work problems. She pointed out that her past reviews were positive and that he hadn't previously mentioned any concerns. When he refused to alter the evaluation, she stated that she disagreed with the review, wouldn't sign it, and requested a meeting with the department manager. Her supervisor then backed down and improved the review. Still angry and offended, Sandy became determined to find another job.

What can you do if you think you're being discriminated against because of your hidden disability? First, document carefully any uncomfortable experiences with your boss or others. Request in writing to have meetings with your supervisor and/or higher up managers. If you have a union, of course, seek help through your shop steward and file a grievance. Utilize any other resources within your company, (e.g., employee assistance programs).

If you can't find help within your organization, consider filing a complaint with a governmental agency. You'll need to consider the pros and cons of this decision since you may face further harassment if you complain. Evaluate all of your options including whether to stay or leave. If you decide to complain, you have two options: 1) contact an attorney and file a lawsuit or 2) file a complaint under the Americans with Disabilities Act.

The ADA and Your Rights on the Job

The Americans with Disabilities Act (ADA) 42 U.S. Code 12101 is a federal law that protects workers from discrimination because of a physical or mental disability that substantially limits a major life activity.

The ADA specifically names a number of conditions that are covered, such as AIDS, cancer, emotional illness, diabetes, and heart disorders. Many other conditions can be covered if the person can prove that the condition restricts a major life activity. Persons with short-term conditions such as being pregnant or breaking a bone are not covered.

According to the ADA, private employers, employment agencies, and labor organizations with fifteen or more workers must make "reasonable accommodations" for workers with disabilities who are competent to

Continued on next page

perform their jobs, unless such accommodations cause the employer undue hardship.

Under the ADA, you have the right to request that reasonable accommodations be made, including:

- modifying facilities such as workstations and rest rooms

- restructuring job responsibilities

- receiving unpaid leave for medical treatment

The ADA also requires that workers have the right to the same opportunities and status as other employees, including salary increases and job promotions. You also have the right to the same health coverage and fringe benefits as those without disabilities.

You have the right to file a complaint with a state or federal enforcement agency. Not all states have special agencies, however. To find out whether your state has a designated agency, contact your state's labor department or attorney general's office. The Equal Employment Opportunity Commission (EEOC) enforces the ADA on the federal level. To find out where your local EEOC office is located, call 1-800-669-3362. The federal office address and phone number: EEOC, 1801 L Street, NW, Washington, D.C. 90507. 1-800-669-3362 (general information and publications), 1-800-800-3302 (TDD), 202-663-4110 (fax). Since there are strict time limits around filing complaints, make sure to file one in a timely manner (Repa 1996).

Coping with Difficult Co-Workers

When Andrea's co-workers discovered that she was on sick leave and recently diagnosed with CFIDS, they volunteered to bring her work at home, asked management for permission to loan her their sick leave, and sent a bouquet of flowers. When Cindy, another CFIDS sufferer, was home ill, several co-workers complained to the manager that CFIDS was nothing more than an overreaction to stress.

Your co-workers may be supportive like Andrea's or resentful like Cindy's. Or you might find people relatively neutral, just going about their business as usual. Perhaps some co-workers are sympathetic and others not. There are several factors at play: Some co-workers may just be more understanding than others. Your good friends may come to your aid faster than the office backbiter. Also, the work environment plays a crucial role. If co-workers feel they're treated well by management, they can often adjust to special situations. But if workers feel oppressed, they may take their frustration out on you.

Here's a list of common reactions by co-workers. Check any that fit for your workplace:

_____ Disbelief: People question whether you're really disabled.

_____ Resentment: Co-workers are angry that you're getting extra breaks or a new workstation.

_____ Worried: They might be overly solicitous, making you feel weak or helpless.

_____ Intrusive: People ask too many nosy questions about your health.

_____ Supportive: Co-workers are genuinely concerned.

_____ Ambivalent: Some days people are supportive; other days you overhear pejorative comments about you. Or some people are accepting while others are not.

_____ Confused: Many people are unfamiliar with hidden disabilities and make insensitive comments out of ignorance.

After reviewing your answers, you'll have a better idea of the challenges ahead. You'll also learn what you need to do next. You may have to set limits with people who are asking too many questions. And if you're facing hostility, speak with the person and, if that doesn't work, to your supervisor.

What you can do to maintain your dignity at work if others resent you or question your condition:

- Pick your battles. It's not worth responding to every comment. However, if there's a pattern of hostility, take action.

- If possible, speak with the person one-on-one. Invite the co-worker to lunch. Say politely, but firmly, "I've valued our relationship. I think that we've been up front with each other before. So I want to let you know that I sense that my illness feels like a burden to you. But it frustrates me when you say that my migraines are all stress related."

- Set limits with overly solicitous co-workers, thanking them for their concern but emphasizing that you want to focus on your work, not your illness, at the workplace.

- Express appreciation to those who've shouldered extra responsibility.

- Offer to help co-workers in any way you can. It will reduce resentment if you offer, for instance, to bring mail to the mail room, photocopy for others, or take minutes at a meeting.

- Don't personalize the comments of others. Your co-worker may be burned out and taking it out on you.

- Be aware of your own resentment or envy by checking in with yourself several times a day. You may be envious that others are not afflicted with a hidden disability. Make sure that your own attitude is not creating friction with co-workers.

- Recognize that some people's thoughtless comments come from misinformation rather than insensitivity. If this is the case, you can use their remarks as a springboard for talking about the realities of having a hidden disability.

- If people persist in being tactless or inappropriate, document all behavior and comments and consider speaking with your supervisor if you think he or she will be supportive.

Managing Clients' Concerns

In addition to coping with difficult bosses and co-workers, you might also be contending with worried clients or patients. If your job involves frequent client contact, your hidden disability might affect clients as well.

Consider Jennifer's predicament. A thirty-one-year-old accountant, Jennifer was diagnosed with ulcerative colitis a year ago and had been hospitalized twice, each time for about a week. Her last hospitalization was at the height of tax season. When she returned to work, she faced not only harried co-workers and bosses but anxious clients. Some clients were understanding and patient, while others were demanding or even angry. Jennifer worked over seventy hours a week to keep up, suffered another attack, and had to go out on disability leave.

It's hard enough to work when you're ill, exhausted, and in pain. The added stress of clients' demands and impatience can send you over the edge. In certain jobs, such as accounting or law, where deadlines abound and clients are paying high fees, it may be impossible to maintain the frenetic pace.

Those of you in the helping professions face special challenges. If you're a counselor or therapist, your clients may see you as their emotional anchor. When you take time off, clients feel angry, abandoned, or insecure. If you return to work with a special back cushion or wrist brace, you may face a barrage of anxious questions.

If you're a nurse, doctor, or other kind of health professional, it may be hard to care for sick patients when you're struggling with your own fears about illness. Hearing about catastrophic health problems can be threatening, as you try not to worry excessively about your condition. Some patients may have unrealistic expectations of you being a pillar of health, which can add more stress.

Managing your health while dealing with needy clients is essential. Here are some suggestions:

- Recognize your limitations. While some clients may expect a lot from you, accept that you're only one person. The term "wounded healer" has been coined to recognize that even helpers are human, subject to illness and other difficulties.

- Develop realistic expectations for yourself and your work. If you used to call clients from home, consider curtailing or reducing this.

- Set limits. While clients may pressure you to do more, you'll need to sometimes say "no."

- Notice if you feel guilty when refusing the requests of others. Remind yourself that you're doing the best that you can. It's not your fault that you have a hidden disability; you have no reason to feel guilty.

- Be assertive. If clients make insensitive remarks like, "You don't look disabled to me," you'll need to find a way to respond assertively yet tactfully, for instance, "Thanks, I'm glad I look fine. There are actually many medical conditions that are disabling even if the person looks okay."

- Maintain your privacy. Don't feel obliged to share details of your condition with your clients. However, you may need to briefly reassure them that you're taking care of yourself.

When You Can't Work

There may come a time when you need to take a temporary or even permanent leave from the work world. Perhaps you've cut back your hours, requested special accommodations like a new chair, and/or worked at home. Yet, continued pain, fatigue, or illness signals that your body needs more rest.

Along with the financial stresses of not working, you face emotional strains as well. Having unstructured time can make you uneasy. You miss the daily contact with co-workers. You have to explain to others why you're at home. You lose the identity of being a worker and may question your value and worth. If another person is providing financial support, you may feel uncomfortable being financially dependent.

You may also feel relieved to not work. There's finally time to rest and recuperate. You get a break from difficult bosses and co-workers. You won't have to explain for the umpteenth time why you look well but feel ill. Not working offers you time to contemplate your life and reconsider your current direction.

In short, leaving work is a mixed bag. You may spiral into depression, or you may feel reenergized. Being home can be liberating or frightening. Here are some ways to alleviate anxiety and optimize your time off:

- Take one day at a time. There may be no way to predict when you'll return to work. Needless worry only drains you.

- Structure your day. If possible, read books, listen to music, rent videos, sit outside, stretch if you can, talk to friends, "chat" with people on the Internet. Be wary of falling into the trap of watching daytime television, which can be depressing.

- Remind yourself of your value even if you're not working. Make a list of your positive traits, for instance, "I'm a good listener," and "I'm honest." Post this list in a visible place, like the refrigerator.

- Learn something new. Buy cassettes of a foreign language, draw, listen to a book on tape. Go to the library and take out books on art. This will help you feel you're being productive while recuperating.

- Rest. Remember that your body needs time to heal. Sleeping late and napping help your body recover. However, be aware of overdoing it. For some conditions, inactivity can exacerbate symptoms. Talk to your health care professional for a more specific recommendation, and always take into account your own instincts regarding your needs.

- Reduce stress. Avoid reading upsetting articles in the paper and turn off the evening news. Do something relaxing before bed to help you sleep.

- Minimize contact with negative people. Invite more positive people into your life.

- Turn to sources of inspiration, such as poetry, books, videos, and, if desired, spiritual practices like meditation or prayer.

What Help Are You Entitled To?

If you've made the decision to take time off of work, you should know your legal rights. The Family and Medical Leave Act (FMLA) offers one option for taking time off when you're too ill to work. If you meet certain criteria, you may be eligible to take up to twelve weeks off of unpaid leave. Most employers are required to authorize the leave, allowing you to return to your current job or a comparable one at the same salary.

The drawback of the FMLA is that the leave is unpaid. But you may have sick leave or vacation time from which to draw. Some states offer disability leave that will pay a percentage of your salary. (You can check with your local unemployment office or local library to see whether your state has disability leave.)

If your health condition is job-related, you may be eligible for workers' compensation. For instance, if you hurt your back on the job, workers' compensation will pay your medical bills and your salary while you recover. However, eligibility can be tricky if you have a preexisting medical condition. For information, contact your local workers' compensation office.

Other assistance you may qualify for includes:

- Unemployment Insurance: In most states, you can only collect unemployment if you are presently physically and mentally capable of working. Also, you have to have lost your job through no fault of your own. Call your local unemployment insurance office for details.

- Food Stamps: This program may help when you're not working or working very few hours. While regulations are often in flux, you generally don't have to be on any other kind of public assistance. Your local county social services agency will generally have information on applying for food stamps.

- Supplemental Social Security Income (SSI): This program provides financial help to people disabled by mental or physical conditions with very low income. You don't need to have paid into the Social Security system. Eligibility requirements are quite strict. Call your local Social Security office for more information.

- Medicare: This medical insurance program covers disabled, as well as elderly, people. As with SSI, it can be hard to qualify. For information, call 1-800-952-8627.

- Social Security Disability Insurance: This program covers workers whose mental or physical disability has lasted more than twelve months and who have paid a certain amount of money into Social Security. Your children may also be eligible for dependents' benefits. The process takes several months but emergency funds may be available. Also, the application process is rigorous, and many people are turned down the first time. Contact your local Social Security office for information.

- Vocational Rehabilitation: While vocational rehabilitation doesn't offer financial assistance, it can help you to obtain retraining in another line of work if your disability prevents you from performing your usual job. To qualify, you'll need to show medical documentation about your condition. Contact your local vocational rehabilitation office (Repa 1996).

Looking for Work

After a period of unemployment, you may be ready to enter the work force—or you may be forced to work because of financial pressures. Or perhaps you're working now, but you've decided to switch jobs. Looking for work under the best of situations is a time-consuming and arduous process. Add to this the pressures of having a hidden disability and the process can feel monumental.

The best way to handle the job search without becoming overwhelmed is to break it down into small, manageable tasks. First, figure out what type of work would suit you. Do research in the library or over the Internet and speak

The Family and Medical Leave Act (FMLA)

The FMLA is a federal law that enables employees to take up to twelve weeks of unpaid leave within twelve months for the medical needs of self or family or for the birth/adoption of a child. The medical leave can be broken up over a year's time or taken all at once. The law penalizes employers who demote or terminate employees who take a lawful leave of absence during this time. Employees can take leave to care for other family members, such as children, grandchildren, parents, or spouses (there is no coverage for domestic partners). You can also use the leave for your own health problems. Problems covered include a broad range of physical or mental disabilities. The law doesn't cover transient medical conditions, such as headaches other than migraines, colds and flues, minor ulcers, or dental work. Also excluded are routine medical or dental visits.

The FMLA includes private and public companies with fifty or more workers. You must have worked for 1,250 hours, or about twenty-four hours per week, during the year before the leave. Certain categories of employees are excluded from coverage, including the highest paid 10 percent of employees; teachers must take their leave at the end of a teaching period.

You can complain within two years after your employer violates the act or within three years if you believe your employer has sought to retaliate against you for asserting your rights under the law. To file a complaint, contact the U.S. Department of Labor. Consult your telephone directory under U.S. Government, Department of Labor, for a local office near you. Your state may also have a family leave statute. You can then file a complaint with this state agency. Contact your state's labor department or the state attorney general's office to see whether your state has family and medical leave protection. You can also file a lawsuit against your employer (Repa 1996).

to people in similar jobs. Ask yourself whether you can be successful at this job with your hidden disability. If you don't feel like it's feasible, you may want to enroll in a career development workshop at a local college or consult a vocational counselor who specializes in career changes.

You'll next want to figure out where you'd like to work. Are there certain companies or agencies that are known for being worker-oriented and humane? Again, doing research and speaking with others are vital. If it's hard for you to do research, enlist others to help. Perhaps a friend can brainstorm with you about possible jobs. Another person can pick up applications for you or drive you to interviews. If friends can't help, call a local volunteer center and see whether someone there can assist you.

Prepare for job interviews beforehand. Many people regard interviewing for jobs as about as appealing as having a root canal. Yet, there are ways to make interviewing less distasteful. One is to gain confidence through practice. Realize that your first interview in a while may feel more awkward than the third or fourth one. Ask a friend to help you answer questions with confidence.

Prior to the interview, investigate the company. Learn about its products, its history, its staff. This will allow you to ask informed questions. Find out as much as possible in advance about what the job entails. Some companies will mail you a job description and a brochure about the organization upon request.

Realize that the person interviewing you is often nervous, too, especially if there's more than one person in the room. He or she may feel pressure to ask innovative questions or appear self-confident. You're probably not the only anxious one! And remember, you're interviewing them, too; you're checking out whether you want to work there. Prepare a few questions in advance to ascertain how much you even want this particular job.

Should you reveal information about your health problem during the job search process? On the one hand, the law is on your side. Along with protecting your rights on the job, the Americans with Disabilities Act (ADA) safeguards you against discrimination during job searches if you're able to do the work with reasonable accommodations. The ADA prevents employers from asking about your medical history or requiring preemployment physicals. Thus, technically you should be able to discuss your special needs without risking the job.

Yet, in reality, it's hard to actually prove that you were discriminated against during the interview process. If you weren't hired, the employer can offer vague reasons like, "The other candidate had more experience," or, "The other person fit in better." Therefore, think long and hard before talking about your hidden disability prior to a job offer.

There are benefits to disclosing in advance: You'll find out the potential employer's attitudes toward health problems, you can find out about their special accommodations, and you won't worry about being later discovered. But there are considerable risks, too, the main one being that the employer may choose someone else. Also, if you get the job, you won't have the choice to maintain your privacy about your hidden disability. You may wonder whether future bosses at the same workplace will harbor resentment about your special needs.

If you do decide to discuss your hidden disability, it's probably wise to wait until you have a job offer, preferably one in writing. Then you can notify your new employer that you have some special needs that require accommodating. The risk is that your supervisor may feel misled since you didn't tell him or her beforehand.

Given that there's no risk-free decision about disclosing, avoid making a blanket decision; consider each job separately. If you have serious reservations about disclosing, take the conservative approach and wait. You can always inform them later on, but, once the cat's out of the bag, it's too late for privacy. Also, consider whether you're looking for employment out of choice or because of financial necessity. If you have the financial stability to take more risks, it may be easier for you to make the decision to disclose information about your hidden disability.

Reminders

You have value and worth apart from your work identity.

Give yourself credit for working while being ill or in pain.

You're not superhuman. Maintain realistic expectations for yourself. Heed the signs of burnout.

It's a personal decision whether to disclose or not. Both involve risks.

Reduce work stress as much as possible.

If you have to take a leave of absence, realize that this may be difficult. Try to engage in meaningful activities, make time to rest and recuperate, and keep your anxiety level low.

When you interview for jobs, recognize that this process is generally stressful. Prepare in advance, and consider carefully the pros and cons of disclosing your hidden disability.

PART II

Surviving and Thriving:
Tools for Healthy Living

CHAPTER **8**

Rebuilding Self-Esteem

I'm really reluctant to tell anyone that I have multiple chemical sensitivities. Most people think I'm crazy or I'm making the whole thing up to get sympathy. Sometimes I think: Maybe they're right. Maybe I am just a neurotic mess.

—Irene, age thirty-two

A hidden disability depletes your self-worth. Previously, you may have felt good about your skills and activities. Your identity was intact: You were a parent or an engineer or an athlete. An illness threatens to rob you of your identity and sense of competency. You wonder: Who am I? If I'm sick all the time, what good am I to anyone? Like Irene, you may be even questioning your sanity.

Given that your health problem is hidden, you're vulnerable to waves of self-hate. You're coping with skepticism or even downright ridicule from others. They admonish you to try a new pill or practice positive thinking. When your symptoms don't disappear, you feel like you're failing them and yourself. Being overwhelmed by an invisible problem that waxes and wanes can feel diminishing. Your self-esteem can plummet.

Self-esteem problems are not confined to people with hidden disabilities. Given the plethora of psychology books on the subject, it's safe to say a great many people suffer from low self-worth. Perhaps you, too, have struggled throughout your life to counteract negative messages about yourself from the past. Irene, for instance, grew up with highly critical parents who chastised her if she got any grades lower than an A. She worked hard over the years to give herself credit and to appreciate her strengths. But developing multiple chemical sensitivities (MCS) seemed to have wiped out those years of progress and left her feeling ashamed and damaged.

Physical problems, like MCS, elicit doubt and questions by others. The stigma may be even more pronounced if your disability is psychological. Announcing to a date that you're on medication for bipolar disorder can lead to a variety of reactions, from disbelief ("But you look normal") to aversion ("I don't think I can handle that") to ignorance ("A friend of a friend is bipolar, and he went to a psychic healer and is off all medications"). It would be difficult for any person to withstand such reactions without his or her self-esteem taking a nose dive.

To feel good about yourself while living with a hidden disability is not an easy task. It means looking within, not without, for validation. If you depend on others around you to restore self-esteem, your hold on self-worth will be tenuous at best. People vary in their ability to be accepting and steadfast; one day your partner may be supportive and the next day express impatience. To handle the rigors of a hidden disability, you need a central core of self-esteem. This chapter discusses what this healthy center is and provides steps for how to rebuild it.

What Is Self-Esteem?

Savannah, age five, is assembling Legos as her mother enters the room. Glowing, Savannah boasts, "Look, Mommy! I'm making an airplane!" Even at this young age, Savannah displays qualities of self-esteem: She's playing happily alone, she's focusing on a task, and she's proudly showing off her accomplishment. Whether her mother reacts with praise or judgment to these type of situations can have a lasting impact on her self-esteem.

Even when you grow up, there's still a five-year-old inside of you yearning for approval and braced for criticism. All children start with vast reservoirs of self-esteem. They love to exhibit their newly acquired skills and talents. But if parents and other significant people are harsh and punitive, children turn on themselves.

You may have struggled during your life to combat a ruthless self-critic. Your inner critic may be your constant companion. Developing a disability where you look outwardly healthy but experience incapacitating pain or fatigue can erode your self-esteem even further. Yet it is possible to build or rebuild self-love and kindness. In fact, it's essential to your emotional and physical well-being.

The first step in restoring self-esteem is to recognize what it consists of. Following is a list of statements that reflect self-worth. It can be helpful to also see whether your self-esteem has dropped since developing a hidden disability.

One way to assess this is to do the test twice, once to record your self-esteem prior to becoming ill and once to evaluate it now. If significantly low self-esteem preceded your developing a hidden disability, you may need professional help to combat feelings of unworthiness. Check off any statements that you feel apply to you:

_____ I am a worthwhile person regardless of my having a hidden disability.

_____ I love myself.

_____ I feel lovable.

_____ I am capable.

_____ I can say no when I need to.

_____ I deserve to be happy.

_____ I deserve to be treated well.

_____ I set limits with people who denigrate my hidden disability.

_____ I feel good about my accomplishments.

_____ I don't seek a lot of approval.

_____ I'm not particularly concerned about what other people think of me.

_____ I don't need a lot of reassurance.

_____ I feel good about my life.

_____ I admire myself for living with the challenges of a hidden disability.

_____ I'm doing the best I can.

_____ I'm attractive.

_____ I associate with people who give me love and respect.

Now review your answers. If you've checked most of these statements, your self-esteem has remained high. However, if you checked few responses, you'll want to focus on feeling better about yourself.

Self-Esteem Busters

Keith, a thirty-year-old systems analyst, was an athlete and world traveler prior to developing Crohn's disease, an intestinal disorder. After a year with the illness, Keith lost thirty pounds, became sedentary, and switched to part-time employment. Not only did his body suffer, but also Keith was crippled by self-loathing. Repulsed by his skinny frame and gaunt face, he wouldn't date. He

Signs of Low Self-Esteem

Here are some common indicators of low self-esteem:

- putting yourself down
- being overly apologetic for your actions
- not standing up for yourself
- feeling worthless and unlovable
- blaming others for problems in your life
- feeling numbed out
- engaging in unhealthy behaviors, such as unsafe sex, addictions, overeating, or overspending
- feeling helpless and powerless
- second-guessing most of your decisions
- doubting your judgment
- seeking validation from others
- rejecting compliments
- not living up to your potential
- remaining in destructive relationships
- doubting your hidden disability
- constantly comparing yourself unfavorably to others
- feeling ashamed much of the time
- feeling inadequate

infrequently called his friends, assuming they wouldn't be interested in seeing him anyway. Keith spent most of his days watching television and smoking marijuana, which, in turn, made him feel even worse.

Keith was suffering from severe low self-esteem precipitated by his hidden disability. Before becoming ill, he was self-assured and independent. Without the activities that gave his life meaning, Keith felt worthless. Negative thinking and self-hate sent him spiraling downward into depression and despair.

Was it Crohn's disease or his reaction to it that sabotaged feelings of self-worth? While it's difficult to live with a painful and debilitating disease, Keith was compounding his misery with self-hate. He was making assumptions about how others felt about his disability. He assumed that women would find him unattractive. He was smoking pot to numb out. (While there's been much controversy about the medical uses of marijuana, it's beyond the scope of this book to argue the pros and cons. Our concern here is not smoking marijuana as an analgesic, but rather as a way to numb out and withdraw from life.) These negative thoughts and behaviors were eroding what remained of Keith's fragile self-esteem.

To rebuild self-esteem, these destructive thoughts and actions—what we call "self-esteem busters"—need to be recognized and challenged. While acknowledging that living with a hidden disability would take a toll on anyone's self-esteem, determine whether you're making yourself feel even worse. You'll also want to identify any dysfunctional behaviors which, in turn, only lower self-esteem even more, trapping you in a vicious cycle.

The following sections describe some common self-esteem busters, as well as providing remedies.

Distorted Thinking

Let's take a look at some typical moments in Keith's day. He wakes up and thinks, "Another crappy day. I don't even want to get up." He drags himself out of bed and goes into the kitchen. He thinks, "If I eat cereal, my intestines will act up." Instead he has a banana, but worries the whole time that it will bring on an attack. Keith thinks about calling his friend, Ed, who keeps leaving messages on Keith's machine. Keith reconsiders: "Ed's probably sick of hearing about my problems." He spaces out in front of the TV and lights up a joint.

Keith's distorted thinking engenders more unhappiness than his intestinal pain which had been absent so far that day. Rather than enter the day with some confidence and hope, he assumes that he'll be in pain. He anticipates that his friend will reject him, so doesn't call. His thoughts bring on self-defeating behaviors, such as social isolation and marijuana use, that, in turn, creates more self-loathing.

Can you relate to Keith? You also may be making assumptions about your life that are harsh and pessimistic. Such negative thinking has disastrous consequences for your mental outlook and self-esteem. Yet the process often occurs automatically; you're not even aware of how you routinely scuttle your efforts and spoil your day. Here's an example of how the vicious cycle of negative thinking works:

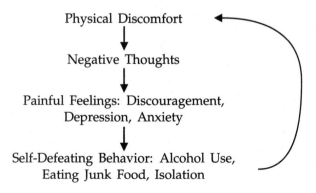

Physical Discomfort

↓

Negative Thoughts

↓

Painful Feelings: Discouragement, Depression, Anxiety

↓

Self-Defeating Behavior: Alcohol Use, Eating Junk Food, Isolation

The solution lies in interrupting this automatic thought process by first becoming aware of it. Following are some of the most common types of distorted thinking. Note the ones that sound familiar to you.

Catastrophizing

This means assuming the worst, for example: "My stomach hurts. I'm in for days of nonstop pain." Try the following suggestions for combating catastrophizing:

- Remember that very few of your worst fears ever come true.

- Realize that worrying about worst-case scenarios won't prevent them from happening; it just produces needless stress.

- Substitute accurate language. For example, "My stomach hurts. It may just be a momentary discomfort. There's no way of predicting. I'll just relax and take a deep breath."

Personalizing

This is when you tend to take things personally, for instance, assuming responsibility for other people's behavior and actions. For example, "John is grumpy today. He's probably sick of dealing with me."

If this sounds familiar, try the following suggestions for combating personalizing:

- Remind yourself that you aren't responsible for how other people react and think. For example, John may be feeling unwell because of a problem in his own life.

- Challenge your assumption that John doesn't want to deal with you. How do you know?

- Substitute accurate language. For example, "John's probably in a bad mood today. I don't know whether or not it has anything to do with our interactions."

Mind Reading

Mind reading is when you are imagining that you know what other people are thinking. For example, "Even though she hasn't said as much, I know my doctor thinks I'm a hypochondriac."

Try the following suggestions for combating mind reading:

- Remember that no one knows what another person is thinking or feeling.

- Ask the person directly to share his or her thoughts.

- Substitute accurate language. For example, "I don't know how my doctor views me."

Filtering

This is the process of only believing or hearing the negative part of the picture. For example, "Jay said he's busy on Saturday. He's probably going to break up with me."

Try the following suggestions for combating filtering:

- Ask yourself, "Am I correctly and completely representing this event?"

- Write down something positive from the situation that you may be ignoring.

- Substitute accurate language. For example, "Jay said he had a good time after our last date, but that he was busy on Saturday. Hopefully he'll call when he's free."

Generalizing

This is the act of making global statements or predictions. For example, "That woman I went out with once never returned my calls. No one will ever want me."

Try the following suggestions for combating generalizing:

- Notice your use of words like "never" and "always," which are generally inaccurate and lead to discouragement and self-depreciation.

- Recall a positive experience when the feared event did not happen, for instance, when a person responded positively to you.

- Substitute an accurate statement. For example, "Even if she doesn't want a second date, I imagine someone else will."

All-or-Nothing Thinking

This is believing that life has to turn out a certain way and that there's no middle ground. For example, "Either I get better or my life is ruined."

Try the following suggestions for combating all-or-nothing thinking:

- Remind yourself that boxing yourself in with absolutes is a recipe for misery.

- Choose to feel some satisfaction even when you're struggling; for instance, appreciate small pleasures like the sight of a blue jay, a smile from a stranger, or the comfort of a favorite blanket.

- Substitute accurate language. For example, "I hope that I get better. But I'll strive to enjoy my life no matter what."

Minimizing

This is the act of downplaying your achievements and successes and/or disregarding the positive events that are occurring. For example, "I've done nothing with my life since I developed this illness."

Try the following suggestions for combating minimizing:

- Write down at least three accomplishments from your day. They can be anything from getting up even though you're depressed to doing stretches for exercise. Review this list when you're minimizing.

- When someone compliments you, notice if you discount it. Rather than disqualify a positive comment, simply say, "Thank you."

- Substitute accurate language. For example, "I've done a lot since I've been ill. I've been handling pain, coping with flack from others, and still taking care of my kids."

"Shoulds"

Keith chooses to take a new medication for his Crohn's disease. The drug doesn't relieve his symptoms and instead gives him a headache. He lambastes himself, "I should never have tried this medication! Now I've got a headache on top of everything else."

In effect, Keith is subjecting himself to "shoulds." By second-guessing his decision, he undermines his ability to trust his judgment. After a while, he feels paralyzed when making any decision, however small.

It's common to bombard yourself with shoulds when you're living with a hidden disability, because you feel out of control. Some people assume that you did something wrong to end up in pain or sick, and they aren't afraid to let you know it. And it's easy to believe that if only you did something right you'd recover. By falling into the trap of shoulds, you may cling to the notion that there must be a simple solution to your health problem.

You do yourself no favor, however, by scrutinizing your every move. While it's painful to accept the reality of having a hidden disability, falling back on shoulds is destructive. As you strive for better health, you need to make hard choices and take risks. Some of these decisions will pay off, while you may regret others. Your task is acknowledging that you don't have complete control over your disability while, at the same time, not giving up the hope of improved health.

Counteracting this type of distorted thinking means seeing your life realistically and acting with compassion toward yourself. Here are some suggestions:

- Remember that no one is omniscient. It's unfair to expect yourself to make the perfect choice and predict the future.

- See mistakes as learning experiences, not character defects. Ask yourself, "What can I learn from this choice?"

- Keep in mind that every person can only control so much in life; then you have to work on letting go.

- Try this technique: When you hear yourself using shoulds, interrupt the thought. Substitute instead, "Here I go again with the shoulds. I'm going to stop this and let myself be human."

Inner Critic

Do you call yourself names, such as "stupid," "weak," "a failure," or "fat"? Do you ruthlessly condemn your skills and abilities? Is it hard to find anything you like about yourself? If so, your "inner critic" may be terrorizing your life and judging your every move. Perhaps you've always lived with a critical voice. You may have internalized the attitude of a nit-picking parent. And now that you've developed a hidden disability, that voice may be blaring with self-recriminations.

One reason why you may be so hard on yourself is to shield you from anticipated put-downs from others. If you worry that friends and family will attack you, you may be inclined to "protect" yourself by hurting yourself first. Then if someone you care about inquires, "Are you still trying that nutty macro-biotic diet?" you're protected from feeling as offended and bruised.

You also may have never forgiven yourself for developing a hidden disability in the first place. You may feel furious, believing that your life is ruined and your potential squashed. You continue to rage at yourself as a form of punishment. Yet this self-condemnation serves no useful purpose. In fact, you only compound your misery. A much gentler approach is to let yourself off the hook for being human. Put your errors in perspective, and don't tolerate your inner critic tyrannizing you. Here are some effective ways to tame your inner critic:

- When you notice that you're beating yourself up for some infraction, ask yourself: "Would I talk to a friend or even a stranger the way I'm talking to myself?" If the answer is no, realize that it isn't okay to condemn yourself in this way, no more than it would be acceptable to treat someone else in this manner.

- Don't allow your critic to operate unchallenged. Record your critical voice in a notebook and talk back to it. For instance, if you call yourself a loser, write this down. Then combat this statement with, "I'm not a loser! I'm struggling with a hidden disability and it's not easy. But I'm doing the best I can, and I'm still a good person."

- In this same notebook, create a compliments page. When someone pays you a compliment, write it down. Review these compliments several times a week.

- Understand the motivation of your inner critic. At the heart of every self-criticism is a genuine concern that has been misdirected. For instance, your inner critic may be trying to prevent you from becoming more disabled. Find out how your inner critic wants to help and then focus that caring energy in a positive way.

- Here's an effective visualization. Imagine a loving and supportive being (this could be a real or imagined person, an animal, a guardian angel, etc.). This being offers you unconditional love and respect—regardless of your flaws. Whenever your critic acts up, visualize this being protecting you. Imagine it challenging and successfully defusing your inner critic.

Unhealthy Behaviors

Negative behaviors spring from hopelessness. Perhaps you feel impotent and discouraged after months or even years of trying to defeat your hidden disability. You're in turmoil from living with a misunderstood and puzzling disorder. Your life is on hold, your relationships are strained, and the future appears dismal. Maybe you've stopped even caring. Given this gloomy picture, it's easy to succumb to dysfunctional habits.

Keith, for instance, smoked pot to ease his emotional suffering and to escape. When high, he didn't have to face his sadness and anxiety. Once active and social, he stayed home most days watching anything and everything on television. Keith felt ashamed of his appearance—his skinny physique and deep worry lines—and minimized his contact with others.

While understandable, such behavior is self-defeating. For instance, you drink because you're depressed. Yet drinking erodes your health even further. Also, given that alcohol is a depressant, it flattens your spirits. Then you feel even more despairing. Clearly, it's vital that you interrupt this vicious cycle.

The first step is to identify your unhealthy behavior. Check off all that apply from the list below:

_____ substance abuse

_____ overuse of pain medications

_____ cigarettes

_____ poor eating habits, such as addiction to sugar

_____ overeating or undereating

_____ little or no exercise

_____ overworking

_____ compulsive sexual behavior

_____ inadequate sleep

_____ little or no relaxation

• _____ high-stress lifestyle

_____ toxic relationships

_____ too much TV watching

_____ staying in bed too long

_____ isolating yourself from others

_____ overspending

_____ other unhealthy behaviors: _____

Once you identify your destructive behaviors, ask yourself why you're involved with them. The reasons may be numerous and complicated. Following are some common reasons why you might engage in unhealthy behaviors:

_____ to distract yourself from pain

_____ to distract yourself from uncomfortable emotions

_____ to give yourself pleasure

_____ because you feel deprived

_____ to be with others

_____ to avoid others

_____ to try to feel better physically, if only temporarily

_____ because you feel hopeless and apathetic

_____ to numb out

_____ because of self-hate or self-punishment

_____ because you're angry at others and are taking it out on yourself

_____ to calm yourself down

_____ other reasons: _____

After reviewing the list, consider your main issues. Are you grappling with self-hate? Are you trying to escape? Is it hard for you to relax naturally? Once you've figured out the motivation, you can work toward change. (You may need professional help for chemical dependency or other compulsive behaviors.)

Here's our four-part program to tackle destructive behavior:

1. Start now. Don't come up with a time in the future to start; that day may never arrive. Make a commitment to begin today.

2. Devise a plan. If you need to reduce your sugar intake, write down a meal plan. You might find it helpful to work collaboratively with a friend who also wants to improve his or her diet. Consider attending a twelve-step program, such as Overeaters Anonymous.

3. Substitute positive behavior. It's often futile to try to stop negative habits without introducing healthier alternatives. For instance, if you just eliminate eating sugar, you'll feel deprived. Instead, take a warm bath, go for a walk, call a friend, or read a book whenever you want sugar, but do not allow yourself to have any.

4. Praise yourself for developing healthier habits. Record in your notebook the ways you've tried that day to combat unhealthy behavior. If you've relapsed, figure out what went wrong. Then move on and begin again with a renewed commitment.

Procrastination

Keith needed to make several pivotal decisions. Running low on money, he had to sell his car and purchase a less expensive one. His boss wanted to know whether he'd return to work full-time. Keith also was considering surgery.

Overwhelmed and confused, Keith avoided making any decision. His inner critic was reproaching him that since he was obviously a loser, any choice he made would be doomed to failure. Keith lost faith in his ability to reason well. Eventually these decisions were made for him: The bank repossessed his car, his boss hired someone else full-time, and his intestinal problems worsened so that he felt forced to have the operation.

Keith's fear of disaster impaired his ability to make choices. Ironically, his avoidance was a self-fulfilling prophesy in that new problems were created. Now his perfect credit rating was ruined and his full-time job was gone. Recovery from surgery was prolonged due to his weakened state prior to the operation.

If you are like Keith, you're ignoring the pressures to make immediate decisions. Even small decisions feel overwhelming. Minor choices that are workable then become crises. Or maybe you're deferring to others to make your decisions. But this type of dependency is fraught with problems. By relinquishing control over your life, you're eroding your self-confidence further, as well as being unfair to your loved ones. In addition, you'll eventually resent the other person for controlling your life, especially if you don't like the outcome of his or her choices. Procrastination contributes to low self-esteem because avoidance conveys the message that "I'm not competent to handle the situation."

There are a variety of reasons why you may be procrastinating. See if any of these sound familiar:

_____   You feel hopeless and don't believe that your decisions even matter.

_____   You feel stupid and unable to make reasonable choices.

_____   You pressure yourself to pick the "right" and "perfect" choice.

_____   You're overwhelmed and overloaded.

_____   You tend to deny that you have a hidden disability that requires adapting to the situation.

_____   You feel that others know better than you what you should do.

_____ You feel ashamed to have a hidden disability and guilty about the problems your disability has caused.

_____ You're intimidated by your inner critic. If you make a mistake, you fear you'll never hear the end of it.

_____ You're scared to fail; you already feel like such a failure with this hidden disability.

_____ You don't want to have to take responsibility for a poor choice.

_____ You're worried that you may regret your choice.

_____ You fear that if you make the wrong decision regarding your health, you'll get worse.

_____ You feel cursed.

_____ You're a fatalist, believing that what happens to you is out of your hands.

A close cousin of procrastination is impulsivity. Rather than feel stuck when you have to choose, you make a hurried decision with little consideration of the pros and cons. For instance, your doctor offers you a risky pain medication. Rather than research the side effects, you fill the prescription and down the pills that night.

Both procrastination and impulsivity are two sides of the same coin—serious ambivalence about making a decision. By procrastinating, you put off making a choice. When you're impulsive, you jump into one blindly. Both derive from fear. You're afraid of the aftermath of a wrong decision, so you hesitate. Or you don't want to face the reality of the situation, so you hastily choose. Both styles can lead to unpleasant outcomes.

By being impulsive or by procrastinating, you're practicing a defense mechanism called "avoidance." You'll want to figure out what you're avoiding. If you fear your internal critic, then follow our suggestions for silencing it. If you're crippled with anxiety, you'll want to find ways to lessen anxiety.

Here's a formula for successful decision making: 1) uncover the obstacles to making decisions, 2) challenge any distorted and self-critical thoughts, 3) outline your options, 4) make a plan of action, and 5) back yourself up.

For instance, Keith sought counseling after surgery because he realized that his life was out of control. He had avoided decision making for so long that his savings were depleted. Keith knew the next step was looking for work, but he felt immobilized.

When asked by his therapist why he was apprehensive about looking for work, he responded, "Fear mainly. Fear of not being able to find a job. Fear of screwing up. Fear that people will think I'm weak or weird if they find out about my disease."

His therapist had him challenge his fears and come up with new possibilities:

1. Determine the obstacle: Fear of not being able to do the work.

2. Challenge distorted thinking: "I'm good at what I do. I'm feeling better. Even if I get sick, there are laws to protect me. No one has to know that I have Crohn's disease. There's no reason why, after some training, I can't do the job."

3. Brainstorm options: Telecommuting; working part-time; finding a job close to home; finding one with flexible hours; looking for a supportive environment that isn't overly competitive.

4. Develop a plan of action: Let friends, acquaintances, and former co-workers know I'm looking, update résumé, finding out about web sites on the Internet, call a few headhunters, apply to jobs in the paper.

5. Provide self-support: "I'm doing the best I can. Job hunting isn't the easiest thing in the world. I'm sure I'll find a job after a while."

Following is a worksheet to help you follow these steps to make a decision:

The decision you need to make is: _____

_____

These are the obstacles to making the decision: _____

_____

_____

These are some options: _____

_____

This is your plan of action: _____

_____

_____

These are some supportive reminders to yourself: _____

_____

Self-Esteem Boosters

When you develop a hidden disability, your self-image becomes distorted. You magnify your blemishes and flaws. You reproach yourself for being weak and inadequate. As we've explained, shoring up your confidence means counteracting negative thoughts, relationships, and behaviors. But that's not enough. You also need to learn new skills and fortify inner strength.

Some essential "self-esteem boosters" are assertiveness, optimism, and resiliency. Assertiveness is a skill that you can learn. By becoming assertive, you'll feel more control as you stand up for yourself. Optimism and resiliency are a little different; they're traits that you may or may not have developed during the course of your life. Some researchers even believe that there's a genetic predisposition for these characteristics. Yet even if they are genetically influenced traits, everyone can still become more optimistic and resilient. And you may want to try; numerous studies indicate that people with these characteristics enjoy a higher quality of life, including longevity.

This means that if you have health problems and you're optimistic and resilient, you may rebound from flare-ups quicker. You may recover faster from bouts of depression or anxiety. You can let other people's careless remarks roll off your back more easily. While your health problems may not disappear, you'll likely cope better.

Assertiveness

Courtney, a twenty-year-old woman in the midst of a fibromyalgia flare-up, spends the day in bed. When her husband arrives home and sees her in her nightgown, he scolds her: "Courtney! You shouldn't spend all day in bed! That will only make you worse. You should be up and about." Courtney wants to defend herself but instead bites her tongue and remains silent.

Courtney is showing a typically passive response. She disagrees with her husband and wants to express her viewpoint, but she censors herself. The end result? Resentment toward her husband, shame about her illness, and further stress on her body.

Do you also hold back on verbalizing your opinion? Do you feel too intimidated to stand up for what you believe? Do you then feel frustrated, misunderstood, and discouraged? If so, you likely have a passive style of relating to others.

Or perhaps you're aggressive. If Courtney had blurted out, "What is your damn problem? Don't tell me what to do!" she would be acting aggressively. While she'd feel better temporarily by letting off steam, her outbursts could alienate her husband and make her feel guilty.

In addition to passivity and aggressiveness, there's a third common reaction—passive-aggressiveness. Had Courtney said nothing but "forgotten" to tell her husband that his friend called, she'd be passive-aggressive. This "sneaky" anger would confuse and irritate her husband without opening up any healthy channels of communication.

There's another choice in these types of situations—assertiveness. Being assertive means expressing your opinions and feelings directly without depreciating the other. You support yourself, preserve your dignity, and respect the other person. To gauge your current style, circle the number that best describes how you'd react to these scenarios:

1. An acquaintance tells you, "If you just start doing yoga, your pain will go away." Your response is:

a. You just sit there; no response.

b. "It's easy for you to say!"

c. You change the subject and share, "I heard that your old boyfriend has a new lover."

d. You say, "I know you're trying to help. But I feel criticized by your comments, like I'm not doing enough."

2. Your teenager wants to have a sleep-over that night. You're not feeling well. Your response is:

a. You say okay because you feel like your poor kid has enough to deal with being stuck with an inadequate parent.

b. You scream, "How can you ask me that? You know I've been sick all day!"

c. You say yes but then act grouchy when your child's friends come over.

d. You say, "No. I don't feel well enough today, but let's talk again about arranging it for another day."

3. Your friend calls and tells you a long story about his day. You're exhausted and just can't listen. Your response is:

a. You say nothing and stay on the phone for an hour.

b. You say with obvious irritation, "Can you cut to the chase? I don't feel well."

c. You "accidentally" cut your friend off.

d. You say, "I wish I could talk longer, but I'm not up to it. I'll try to call you tomorrow if I'm better."

4. Your boss asks you to stay late again. She knows that you requested the afternoon off a week ago to go to physical therapy. She says something important came up and you need to stay. This is not the first time such "emergencies" have come up when you have a doctor appointment. Your response is:

a. You say nothing and cancel the appointment.

b. You say with irritation, "You know, I asked a week ago for the time off!"

c. You say nothing and badmouth her later to your co-workers.

d. You say, "I can't stay today. I requested the time off a week ago and you approved it. It's important that I keep my appointment. I'll be glad to take care of the project tomorrow."

Now, review your answers. If you have mostly "A" answers: Your style is passive. You probably feel trampled on by others and contemptuous of yourself. "B" responses reveal an aggressive stance. You have pent-up rage that you're having difficulty controlling. Your relationships with others are likely suffering.

"C" answers show a passive-aggressive style. You sneak your anger in rather than express it directly. This style bewilders and alienates others. "D" responses demonstrate assertiveness. You feel entitled to your feelings. You take care of yourself without devaluing the other person.

Barriers to Assertiveness

By now, you may be enthusiastic about learning some techniques for assertiveness. But first you'll want to figure out why you're unassertive in the first place. Examine the following list, checking any that apply:

_____ You don't want to hurt other people's feelings.

_____ You're scared of not being liked, especially now that you're ill.

_____ You feel guilty if you voice your opinion.

_____ You worry that the other person will abandon you.

_____ You fear others will retaliate.

_____ It's vital that you be liked.

_____ You don't want to be seen as a bitch or a bastard.

_____ You don't want people to be angry at you.

_____ You're so frustrated that you lash out at others.

_____ Since you've become ill, you're impatient and verbally attack others.

_____ You're ashamed of who you are.

_____ Other reasons: _____

Did you check any of the above? If so, you may have certain roadblocks to asserting yourself. Perhaps you've always struggled to assert yourself. It's even harder now that you've developed a hidden disability. You worry that other people will leave you if you don't acquiesce. You feel guilty for being an ill partner or parent. Or maybe you've tended to be aggressive. Now you're so frustrated by callous remarks that it's hard to hold your tongue and respond calmly.

The first step, then, is to feel entitled to being assertive. Read the next section, which discusses the myths and realities about assertiveness. If you believe these myths, you'll want to substitute realities. Most especially, even if you have a hidden disability, remember that you still have a right to your own feelings, attitudes, and opinions. No one has the prerogative to mistreat you or take advantage of you.

Myths and Realities about Assertiveness

Myths:	**Realities:**
Everyone else's needs are more important than yours.	You have a right to put yourself first.
You don't want to hurt other people's feelings.	You have a right to not let your feelings get hurt.
When you get mad, you just tell whoever you're mad at that they are an asshole.	You don't have to demean others to express yourself.
You should never rock the boat, especially now that you're sick.	You have a right to express yourself, even if you have a health problem.
It's not nice to say "no."	You don't always have to be nice. It's okay to set limits.
You should always assert yourself.	You can "pick your battles."

How to Be Assertive

Here are some effective methods for assertiveness. Pay special attention to the tips on body language. If you're saying the right words but, for example, you appear meek and obsequious, your point won't get across effectively.

Presenting Yourself Assertively

Following are some suggestions for assuming an assertive style of communicating:

- Use a strong voice, both audible and clear.

- Make eye contact.

- Keep your head held high.

- Don't slouch; notice your posture.

- Don't apologize.

- Take your time.

- Be courteous and respectful.

- Breathe and try to relax.

"I" Statements

By using the word "I" instead of "you," you take responsibility for your feelings and avoid blaming the other person. Here's an example: Your doctor tells you that stress is the culprit and refuses to order tests to determine the reason for your headaches.

"You" Statement: "Doctor, you just don't understand. You are not being helpful at all!"

"I" Statement: "I know that you're trying to help, and I appreciate it. But I feel disqualified when you keep talking about my stress. It would help a lot if you could instead offer ideas for treatment."

Here's a format to use:

When you did or said: _____

It made me feel: _____

I'd prefer that you'd: _____

Broken Record

With this method, you repeat your point over and over without backing down. So if your doctor urges you to examine your stress, you say, "As I said, Doctor, I feel disqualified when you attribute my symptoms solely to stress. I prefer that we focus on new tests that can rule out medical problems." You continually restate your position.

Staying Focused

When you assert yourself with others, they may change the subject and throw you off course. Don't let them. For instance, if your doctor says, "But you did ask me for a referral to a psychotherapist because you're depressed," you answer, "Yes, but I'm depressed because of my hidden disability. Now, again, I want to focus on whether you can get approval for an MRI."

Fogging

Use fogging when you want to appear to agree with another person while standing your ground.

Doctor: I still think that your depression may be at the root of things.

You: You may be right, but I don't want to consider that until we've eliminated all medical possibilities. Now how long will it take for you to get authorization for an MRI?

Optimism

It's hard to remain hopeful when you have a hidden disability. Even if your personality tends toward optimism, being sick and tired for days on end will challenge the most invincible spirit. Just when you think you're getting better, you relapse. You develop new and disturbing symptoms out of the blue. Your friends and family implore you to "think on the bright side," but you can't figure out what that is.

While being optimistic is no easy task, there are a number of potential payoffs. Optimistic people often bounce back quicker from adversity. In several studies of cardiovascular patients, optimism was linked to longer life span, faster recovery, and fewer medical complications (Goleman 1995). In a study of people who suffered spinal cord injuries, those who were hopeful gained greater levels of physical mobility (Elliot et al. 1991).

Since optimism is often misunderstood, it's important to understand what it is and isn't and what it can and can't do. It's not acting like Pollyanna, being phony and smiling all the time. And optimism doesn't cure disease or prevent illness from happening in the first place. It does mean living life in the present and not jumping to negative conclusions about the future. It's remaining hopeful even when you're experiencing hard knocks. Optimism won't cure your hidden disability, keep you in a perpetual happy state, or eliminate pain. It can, however, help you endure defeats more easily and rebound from flare-ups and callous treatment by others.

To test whether you lean toward optimism or pessimism, choose your most likely responses:

1. You feel the first twinges of pain. You think:

   a. Oh no! I'm always going to be in pain.

   b. This will clear up soon.

2. Your therapist says in almost every session, "I don't think you're getting better because you're benefiting unconsciously from assuming the sick role." You think:

   a. No one will ever understand me.

   b. I'm tired of being blamed for my disability. I'm going to look for a more supportive therapist.

3. Your nurse practitioner diagnoses your condition. You think:

   a. My life is over. I'm totally worthless.

   b. Finally a diagnosis. Now I'm going to find a way to live with this problem.

4. Your partner gets frustrated with you for not doing any housework like you'd planned. You think:

   a. I'm a burden to my partner.

    b. My partner's upset, but I know I did what I could. I need to talk to him (or her) and see what's going on.

5. Your children yell at you when you ask them to turn down the television because your head hurts. You think:

    a. I'm such an inadequate mother; they'll probably always resent me for being sick.

    b. They'll be angry for a while, but they'll eventually understand.

Now, review your answers. Mostly "A" responses reveal a pessimistic style. You feel helpless about events in your life. You view setbacks as crises and disasters. Rather than view difficulties as specific, you assume they're permanent fixtures in your life. Consequently, you're overwhelmed and depressed. While you'll have to do some work to become more optimistic, remember that it is possible for you to change this thought pattern.

If you circled mostly "B" responses, you tend to be optimistic. You're less apt to personalize situations and make harsh judgments against yourself. You view hardships as bearable and manageable. Your optimistic attitude inoculates you against descending into depression and despair.

Acquiring Optimism

Pessimistic thinking is an automatic habit. Perhaps you have been pessimistic most of your life. Or maybe becoming ill has stifled your optimistic disposition. In either case, it is possible to think more positively. Like breaking the habit of smoking, it can be hard to eliminate pessimistic thoughts. But, as millions of ex-smokers can testify, compulsive behavior can be stopped.

Use "the three D's" to interrupt your pessimistic voice: Disagree with your negative voice. Distance yourself from the thoughts by labeling them as pessimistic. Develop positive ways of thinking.

For instance, Charlene, a nineteen-year-old college student diagnosed with Tourette's syndrome, a neurological tic disorder, confided her condition to a close friend. The friend responded, "I heard of someone who had that problem. She switched to a macrobiotic diet and was cured." Charlene's immediate thought was, "Why do I even bother trusting people? They are just going to judge me and give me pat suggestions."

In therapy, Charlene recognized that such pessimistic thinking was making her feel discouraged and alone. She counteracted her thinking using the "three D's" approach:

1. Disagreeing with her pessimism: "How do I know that everyone will judge me? I can't generalize about the entire population."

2. Distancing herself from her pessimism: "I'm being pessimistic again. This doesn't mean that my thoughts are true."

3. Developing more positive ways of looking at her situation: "I'm disappointed that my friend reacted this way, but she's just trying to be helpful. She may need some education about Tourette's syndrome."

Here's a worksheet to help you develop more optimistic thinking:

Event: _____

Pessimistic thought: _____

I'm going to disagree with this thought by reminding myself: _____

_____

I'm going to distance myself from this thought by reminding myself: _____

_____

Positive thoughts that I can replace my pessimistic thoughts with include:

_____

Resiliency

Resiliency is closely related to optimism. Optimism is a positive, hopeful attitude. Resiliency is an inner strength that enables you to recover from setbacks and disappointments. A resilient person perseveres during hard times, never gives up hope, and bounces back time and time again.

Helene, a forty-two-year-old computer analyst, embodies resiliency. When she was diagnosed with Ménierès disease, an inner ear disorder, it was just a year after her divorce. She had just started venturing out more and exploring new activities. Helene was sad and angry at first that she developed this debilitating, chronic problem.

But finally Helene said to herself, "I've had it with being miserable." She learned all she could about the disorder and tried a few alternative treatments. On good days, she'd visit friends, go for walks, and work from home. During flare-ups, she'd stay inside, rest, and play relaxation tapes. Her friends were inspired by her continued warmth and caring even in the midst of pain and illness.

Let's identify the qualities that made Helene resilient:

- A take-charge attitude: After initially being bowled over, she refused to feel like a victim and instead became an informed consumer.

- Ability to grieve: Note that Helene didn't deny her feelings or put on a happy face. She faced her losses, adjusted, and moved on.

- Focus outward: Rather than remain self-absorbed, she kept involved in the world.

- Acceptance: While Helene searched for ways to feel better, she accepted her hidden disability as reality. She optimized her good days and learned to live with her bad ones.

- Practical attitude: Helene experienced her emotions; however, she didn't get mired in them. She focused on finding solutions to her problems.

- Flexibility: She adapted to changing life circumstances.

To see how resilient you are, answer the following questions by circling the answer that best describes your reactions:

I see flare-ups as challenges, not crises. *yes   no*

When I get new symptoms, I'm confident that I can cope. *yes   no*

I accept hardships and setbacks as a part of having a hidden disability.
yes   no

I believe that I can handle anything life throws my way. *yes   no*

If people doubt my symptoms, I don't let it get me down. *yes   no*

I rarely focus on the past or worry about the future. *yes   no*

I've accepted my hidden disability as part of my life. *yes   no*

I've remained as active as possible. *yes   no*

I feel hopeful about the future. *yes   no*

I'm flexible and adapt well to change. *yes   no*

I accept that pain and suffering are part of being human. *yes   no*

If you answered "yes" to nine to eleven questions, consider yourself a resilient person. If you answered "yes" to six to nine questions, realize that you possess some resilient traits and work on acquiring more resilient qualities. If you answered "yes" to five or fewer questions, resiliency isn't playing much of a role among your current coping skills. You may be having trouble coping with your hidden disability. You likely feel pummeled by life and have difficulty recovering from disappointments. But just because resiliency hasn't been your strong suit in the past doesn't mean it can't be in the future. You'll just have to work on it more than you would have had to otherwise.

Developing Resiliency

There are several things you can do to become more resilient. First, realize that you've endured difficulties before. Making a list of problems you've overcome can help remind you. Below, record any hardships during your life and how you survived. Then write down your inner strengths that enabled you to cope. (Remember that you still possess these coping skills and can draw from them at any time.)

Hardships: _____

_____

These are ways that I persevered: _____

_____

I possess these qualities, which help me to cope with adversity: _____

_____

Next, congratulate yourself for living with a hidden disability. Recognize that this, too, takes courage and resiliency. Then take the next step by acquiring new skills to enhance your resiliency. For example, a helpful visualization is imagining having a caring "coach" who helps you through difficult times, reminding you: "You can do it! You've got what it takes." Just as a sports coach encourages his or her team, your inner coach urges you to persevere and remain hopeful.

It also helps to develop a more realistic attitude about life—people get disabilities, things happen in life that you can't change. Feeling victimized and cursed by your set of circumstances will drain you of resources that are better used coping. Remind yourself that life is hard for everyone, although the problems differ.

Another sign of resiliency that you can incorporate into your way of being is to see life predicaments as challenges. As Carlos Castenada has written, warriors tend to see life in terms of challenges, not problems. Imagine yourself as this warrior who has the inner resources to conquer whatever life has in store for you. Finally, collect inspiring articles and stories about other people who have overcome difficult life events. When you feel alone and overwhelmed, read through these articles. Remind yourself that, like the heroes you've read about, you can get through hard times, too.

Reminders

You are not your disability. You are greater than the sum of your physical or emotional limitations.

It's common for your self-esteem to take a beating when you develop a hidden disability.

To feel good about yourself again, look within for support.

If you pummel yourself for being ill, you'll make yourself even more miserable.

You have more inner strengths and tenacity than you've been aware of previously in your life.

Compliment yourself for enduring the hardships of a hidden disability.

Try to feel good about the kind of person you are, and don't focus in on your physical limitations.

You have a right to assert yourself even though you have a hidden disability.

CHAPTER **9**

Strengthening Your Body and Spirit

I never loved my body. But it functioned just fine. I don't like to admit it, but sometimes I hate my body. When my back hurts, I feel furious at it for letting me down.

—Barb, age forty-two, diagnosed
with a herniated disc

When you develop a hidden disability, your body takes a beating—and so does your spirit. Before, your body was your faithful companion, accompanying you on innumerable adventures. Now it can seem as though your body has turned against you. Parts of your body that worked quietly behind the scenes now demand your attention. While you never noticed your knee before, having it ache puts it in the spotlight. You wish you could go back to the days when your body functioned automatically and efficiently.

Like Barb, you may have come to detest your body because you feel betrayed by it. It's preventing you from working, having fun, or just taking care of business. Your self-esteem has likely suffered because your appearance reflects months of deconditioning and physical pain. As Barb explains:

I've never been a beauty queen. I've always struggled to lose fifteen pounds or so. Yet now that I'm sedentary, the weight has piled on. I know that my friends are talking behind my back and wondering why I've porked out. They think I'm lazy and depressed. Maybe I am depressed, but who wouldn't be?

You can get caught in an endless cycle where you reduce exercise because you're in pain, you gain or lose weight, and then any exertion hurts. So you avoid doing exercise, your physical appearance declines further, and the cycle continues. When you can't fit into your clothes and dread buying new ones, your self-contempt rises.

Developing a hidden disability requires adapting to the changes in your looks and abilities. If you reveled in your taut muscles and toned physique, you have to get used to looking differently. Perhaps your complexion has changed or you've experienced hair loss. Any of these shifts—coupled with the normal decline of aging—can evoke shame and self-consciousness. You may go out less and fear meeting new people or bumping into old friends.

When you develop a hidden disability, you go through a process of grieving your old body and trying to accept your new one. You long for a return to your former state. Some of the changes may be temporary, and you can look forward to regaining your former appearance. College sophomore Selena, for instance, was mortified when she suddenly lost all of her body hair, an autoimmune condition called alopecia universalis. After several months, her hair began regrowing as unexpectedly as it had fallen out. Although the condition reversed itself, Selena grieved the loss of the illusion that she had complete control over her body.

In other cases, changes are irreversible. Several years ago, Francine, a forty-two-year-old homemaker, developed scleroderma, a puzzling autoimmune disorder that hardens the skin and internal organs. Her skin became reddened and rubbery. She was embarrassed to go out because people stared. The loss of body function, coupled with appearance changes, plunged her into a state of profound grief.

A hidden disability not only devastates your body; your spirit also takes a battering. Developing a psychiatric or physical disability can shatter your faith in yourself, your world, and your spiritual beliefs. When your friends talk about their recent trip to France, you may wonder, "Why me? Why am I stuck with these problems?" A universe where you have to live with pain and restrictions may not be a place where you want to reside.

While you may not recover your health, it's essential that you try to reclaim your spirit. Your spirit is your aliveness, your life force. Without it, you become emotionally disabled. It takes time to grieve your losses, feel your anger, and adapt to your disability. It's natural to feel lost and confused for a time.

Mending your spirit means remembering that you're essentially the same person you always were. Who you are transcends your physical body; your life force endures under any circumstance. How else can we explain, for example, how some children are terribly abused and yet go on to becoming loving and accomplished adults?

While at times it may seem impossible to thrive while living with a hidden disability, you can. But it takes time, considerable effort, and tolerance of the ups and downs along the way. Accepting that you won't do it perfectly is an important part of your experience.

This chapter offers you some tools for mending your body and spirit. We'll provide suggestions for promoting physical well-being. Your spirit can also be nourished through positive practices, such as altruism and creativity. By nurturing your body and spirit, it's possible to live deeply and fully even if you have chronic pain or illness.

Making Peace with Your Body

Your body helps to define who you are. If you continually rage at your body as unattractive, weak, and inadequate, you'll be saddled with self-hate along with a hidden disability. While it's natural to feel ambivalent about your body and be angry at it sometimes, don't let these emotions consume your life. Making peace with your body is an important step in fostering healing.

How do you make peace with your body when it's let you down and caused you pain? Richard, a fifty-one-year-old attorney, experienced this dilemma. He had a heart attack around his fortieth birthday, after running a race. Once a competitive athlete and workaholic, Richard lived in fear of another heart attack. He worried incessantly and avoided exercise. Richard regarded his body as the enemy with the potential to destroy his life at any time. When Richard's blood pressure remained high, a friend pointed out gently that Richard's unremitting self-contempt might be putting his health at risk.

You may relate to Richard's story, fearing and detesting your body. While these reactions are understandable, it's vital that you shift your perspective. Remaining angry at your body only reinforces feelings of helplessness. Your body is part of you. Finding ways to befriend your body is a difficult—though essential—task.

Remember that your body hasn't meant to hurt you. Sometimes bodies just develop pain and uncomfortable symptoms. Parts wear out. And even though your body feels broken, most of it works. Your back aches but your eyes still see. You may be overcome by fatigue but your heart and lungs are strong. Or maybe you're stricken with a psychiatric disability and yet the rest of your body remains healthy.

The place to start is forgiving your body for causing you suffering. This doesn't mean that you're happy about developing a hidden disability. But it does mean treating your body with understanding instead of hate. Through forgiveness, you cultivate appreciation for what does work. You also recognize that your body is working hard to heal. Cultivating a loving attitude toward your body can go a long way toward mending your body as well as your broken-down spirit.

Use this exercise to help you make peace with your body:

Find a comfortable place to sit and relax. Take a few deep breaths, and calm your body. Next, take a couple of minutes to scan your body from head to toe. As you do this, notice all of the parts of your body that are working fine with no help from anyone. Visualize your eyes seeing, your lungs breathing, your heart pumping blood throughout your system. As you do this, express appreciation to your body. Say, for instance, "I appreciate that my kidneys are functioning." Thank the different parts of your body for working so hard to keep you alive. Say to your body, "I know that you struggle sometimes. But you're doing the best you can. Thank you for your effort."

Tuning In

Sharon, a thirty-four-year-old computer analyst, was diagnosed with carpal tunnel syndrome six months ago. Her doctor, whom she trusted, advised her to wear a wrist splint most of the time. But reading through articles on the Internet, Sharon learned that many professionals discouraged the use of splints, especially while typing. She didn't know whom to believe.

It's common to be offered contradictory advice from various health care professionals. Like Sharon, you might become confused about how to treat your hidden disability. Your doctor may suggest rest while your physical therapist urges exercise. A friend's cortisone injection eliminates her pain while yours has negative side effects. With all the varying opinions, you can become paralyzed with indecision about how to proceed.

The first step is to learn what is helpful for your particular problem. If you have a herniated disc, rest may be in order. But with fibromyalgia, a sedentary lifestyle usually worsens the condition. Migraines are treated with ice, while sinusitis is treated with heat. If you have a diagnosis, it's up to you to become an authority on your problem.

Yet not every disorder can be diagnosed. And even if you have a label for your condition, what works for someone else may make you worse. The key is to tune into what makes you feel better. You are the real expert on your hidden disability. While doing researching and connecting with others can offer you guidance along the way, the journey is your own.

Sharon, for instance, can find valuable information from talking to her doctor, seeking second opinions, and joining a repetitive strain injury support group. But, ultimately, her body is her best guide. If a splint reduces her pain and allows her to work longer on the computer, it may be helpful. If, instead, her wrist is tighter and weaker, Sharon needs to question whether splints are working. Rather than continue to search for a definitive answer from an outside source, Sharon needs to look within.

Paying attention to your body may not be easy. Before you developed a hidden disability, you may have been clearer about the warning signs. When you were exhausted, you figured you were getting a cold and slowed down. If your knee throbbed, you took a break from jogging for a couple of days. Now your pain may be misleading and ambiguous. If you have myofascial pain, for instance, pain may or may not signal an injury. It's hard to know how to treat the pain.

Another hurdle to tuning in is feeling numbed out physically. Perhaps you have always had difficulty being attentive to your body. If you've been sexually or physically abused, you may have blunted your awareness of your body. Or you may have been attentive before, but months or years of physical pain and upsetting experiences with health care providers have rendered you detached. If this is the case, learning what helps and doesn't help your body may be difficult. You may need help to reexperience your body without feeling threatened and unsafe.

There are many ways to tune in to your body and to heed its warning signals. Here are some tips:

- Know that there are no absolutes. What works for one person may be useless or even detrimental to you. Given this, you'll need to take some reasonable risks, which may or may not pay off. Be forgiving and kind toward yourself if you try something that doesn't work.

- Resist the urge to blindly follow other people's advice. If you feel uneasy, trust your instincts. Investigate the pros and cons.

- Learn your body's signals. If you're exhausted after a ten-minute walk, reduce it to five minutes. See if you can slowly build up.

- Take pain and other uncomfortable sensations seriously. If others are dismissing your symptoms as psychosomatic, you may end up ignoring bodily discomfort. Don't do this. Remember that you are your body's owner and, therefore, the best judge of what you need.

- Accept that not knowing is part of living with a hidden disability. If the "experts" can't predict with certainty what will work, how can you expect to always know what's best? Flare-ups are likely an unavoidable consequence of living with chronic pain and illness.

Guidelines for Self-Care

Relating to your body with kindness and tuning in are important—but they're not enough. It's also crucial to introduce healthy habits such as good nutrition, appropriate exercise, and beneficial treatments. Self-care will improve your health and boost your spirits.

To assess your care of your body, answer the following questions:

1. I eat vegetables daily. *yes*   *no*

2. I eat fruit daily. *yes*   *no*

3. I've reduced or eliminated sugar. *yes*   *no*

4. I've reduced or eliminated fat. *yes*   *no*

5. I've reduced or eliminated animal products. *yes   no*

6. I don't smoke. *yes   no*

7. I don't use recreational drugs. *yes   no*

8. I don't drink alcohol (or drink only in moderation). *yes   no*

9. I consume caffeine infrequently or not at all. *yes   no*

10. I'm careful about what I put in my body. *yes   no*

11. I stretch daily as much as I can. *yes   no*

12. I exercise as much as I can. *yes   no*

13. I practice safe sex. *yes   no*

14. I'm careful about not overdoing medications. *yes   no*

15. I drink several glasses of water throughout the day. *yes   no*

16. I feel that, in general, I take good care of my body. *yes   no*

If you checked "yes" for thirteen or more answers, you're taking good care of your body. Fewer than twelve means that you could benefit greatly by improving your self-care. Read on for ideas on how to make changes.

Resistance to Self-Care

You've probably read countless articles about the need to eat right, drink plenty of water, and exercise. You may have resolved to improve your health habits. Yet, after a few days or weeks, you're bingeing on ice cream and potato chips.

The first step in changing habits is understanding why you're resistant. Review the following list and check all that apply:

_____ Nothing seems to work, so I don't even care anymore.

_____ I hate my body; I don't feel like being good to it.

_____ I'm scared to exercise.

_____ Whatever I eat bothers my system, so why bother trying to be healthy?

_____ I'm too weak to give up caffeine or alcohol.

_____ I'm angry at my body. Maybe I want to punish it.

_____ I already feel different. I don't want to stand out even more when I'm with others.

_____ My (partner, friends, etc.) like to party and overeat. They'll think I'm even more neurotic if I bow out.

_____ I already feel so deprived. I don't want to cut out desserts, coffee, etc.

After reviewing your answers, notice the reasons why you're resisting practicing self-care. Are you depressed or angry? Are you frightened to exercise? Do you feel peer pressure? Once you're aware of the hurdles, you can respond. You can work to counteract feelings of depression or anxiety. If you're feeling deprived, you can substitute healthy habits like taking hot baths or getting massages. Rather than viewing changes as deprivation, alter your thinking. View healthy habits as a way of regaining some control over your life.

It may feel overwhelming to imagine making changes. You've got enough to do just to make ends meet and take care of your family. Improving your diet or beginning a stretching program feels like a monumental "should." While it may be important to start changing habits, don't unduly stress yourself about it. Start small. Even restricting sugar for one day is a good start. It's counterproductive to overdo it anyway. Suddenly changing your diet or beginning an aggressive exercise program will overly tax your body. Given that you'll likely fail if you try too much at once, you'll become discouraged as well.

We'll now describe some healthy habits to consider. See which ones sound doable and intriguing. Be aware of overwhelming yourself with pressure about doing it all. Begin slowly and pace yourself.

Exercise

You know that exercise is good for you. But the problem is, how do you do it regularly when you don't feel well? It's easy for others to recommend hiking or biking. But when you're exhausted and achy, even walking up a flight of steps seems impossible.

It's true that exercise can improve your stamina and boost your spirits. Exercise produces natural endorphins that relieve pain and elevate your mood. But exercise can also hurt. If you have a hidden disability, you have to take special care not to overdo it. The chronic fatigue and immune dysfunction syndrome (CFIDS) sufferer may end up exhausted from too much exercise. The person with fibromyalgia may end up with new trigger points and greater discomfort. If you have a repetitive strain injury, you have to guard your body from further strain. Sometimes it may feel like all the extra effort isn't worth the risk of feeling any worse.

Most people with hidden disabilities can exercise. The challenge is to know your limits. Of course, this is easier said than done. One week you can walk a half mile and feel fine afterward. The next week you're laid up in bed for days after taking a shorter walk. Your friend swears that swimming calms her pain. But when you do it, your symptoms flare up.

Exercise is also one of those areas where others may not understand your special needs. Friends may believe that you'll be cured if you just take up some physical activity. They urge you to "feel the burn" but push past the pain. Maybe you consider yourself a wimp if you only walk a few blocks rather than a few miles. Given that your disability is hidden, your tendency may be to ignore the pain in your knees or your exhaustion. But you quickly learn that while pushing past the pain works for some people without health problems, you end up flared up.

Your first task is to accept that you have limitations and unique needs. Even if your disability is undiagnosed, you know intuitively that something is wrong. While a short bike ride may be fine for your friend, this exertion feels like too much for you. Your symptoms are communicating an important message. They're asking for your attention. Ignoring your body's warnings often leads to increased pain and disability. While it may feel embarrassing to have to end early with your walking or swimming partner, you must put your own needs first. If your friend teases or pressures you, explain your needs to him or her. If your friend persists in being unsupportive, find a new exercise companion.

Here are some other suggestions for your exercise program:

- Pay attention to your own body. If your doctor pushes you to immediately begin a rigorous sport, think twice. It's generally best to start slow, especially if you're out of shape. Start with a low-impact form of exercise, like walking or swimming; however, keep in mind that even walking and swimming have their risks. If you're exhausted or in pain, stop. Learn about your body's unique capabilities and limits. Try not to be concerned about what other people think.

- It can be helpful to at first divide up your exercise regimen throughout the day. Rather than walk for twenty minutes straight, start with ten minutes in the morning and ten more in the afternoon. You can do a few minutes of stretching at one point in the day and then stretch again in the evening.

- Consider t'ai chi or yoga as other options. Both are ancient forms of exercise that combine gentle movement, stretching, breathing, and meditation. If you can't attend a class, you can purchase audio or videotapes demonstrating movements. (However, keep in mind that any form of exercise has risks.)

- Give yourself a lot of credit for starting an exercise program. Recognize that there will likely be times when you're not up to exercising. If you suffer a setback, you might have to stop exercising for a while. Try not to become discouraged; when you're ready, begin again.

Healthy Eating

In most cultures food is a major source of pleasure. The choices of restaurants and delectable foods at the market are unlimited. Treating yourself to a succulent meal and dessert is a satisfying reward at the end of the day. Food is also a way of making connections with others. Meeting over dinner, coffee klatches, and family meals foster closeness and intimacy.

Yet, when you have a hidden disability, you often have to restrict your diet. It can seem unfair to have to limit one more part of your life, especially when food is so pleasurable. It's frustrating to have to refuse a slice of cheese-cake or forgo an invitation to a barbecue. You've already given up so much. Yet, if you don't watch your diet, you risk jeopardizing your health.

Nick, a forty-two-year-old man with inflammatory bowel disease, needed to significantly restrict his diet. He'd always loved rich foods and desserts; staying on the special diet felt like torture. He was also embarrassed to refuse pastries and alcohol when he went to parties. Depressed, Nick returned to his regular diet. A serious relapse landed him in the hospital. In therapy, he received help for coping with his considerable grief and anger over having to give up his old way of eating.

Can you relate to Nick? Perhaps you, too, are struggling to eat healthily. While you know that you "should" be careful about what you eat, you sometimes rebel. You end up sabotaging your efforts and then feel guilty and weak. Your reasons for not wanting to change your diet may in fact be hidden and unconscious. Let's take a look at possible reasons why you might resist. Check those statements that ring true:

_____ Sugar is like a drug; I can't stop eating it.

_____ I can't get through the day without caffeine.

_____ Drinking helps me to relax. I'll be uptight without it.

_____ I refuse to give up one more thing.

_____ Maybe the emphasis on healthy eating is overblown.

_____ I'll be miserable on a healthy diet.

_____ Healthy foods don't taste good.

_____ My friends or family will give me a hard time.

_____ I already feel out of place; I don't want to feel even more different.

_____ Nothing helps anyway.

By examining your statements, you can figure out your roadblocks. If you're catastrophizing that your life will be unhappy without french fries and chocolate, of course you'll rebel. If you fear being ridiculed or ostracized by others, it will be harder to change your diet.

After you determine the barriers, the next step is to reframe them in your mind. For instance, Nick could relate to the statement, "I'll be miserable on a healthy diet." He needed to challenge this automatic belief. He came up with the following revision:

> Being on a healthy diet may be hard at first. But this doesn't mean I'll be miserable. In fact, it will feel great knowing I'm controlling my disease. If I can minimize flare-ups, giving up fat and sugar will be well worth it.

It's helpful to turn discouraging self-talk to more positive self-affirmations. Here's a worksheet to use:

Resistance: _____

_____

Revision: _____

_____

Here are some other tips for maintaining a healthy diet:

- If you slip up, don't be unduly harsh or critical with yourself. Just make a renewed commitment to healthy eating.

- Beware of radical diets that require an extreme reduction of certain foods. Follow these only with the assistance of medical professionals.

- Most experts believe that plant-based diets are healthier than ones focused on meat and dairy. Consider reducing your intake of animal products. Make significant changes slowly and carefully. Switching abruptly from a meat-based to a vegetarian diet, for instance, may overly stress your body.

- Eat organic foods whenever possible. If you can, grow some of your own food. Sprouts, for instance, can be grown easily in your kitchen.

- Reduce sugar intake. Even honey and maple sugar have high sugar contents.

- Drink lots of water—but try to avoid straight tap water if possible. Buy bottled water or purchase a filter for your faucet.

- Consider supplementing your diet with vitamins and nutritional supplements. (Some vitamins and herbs have risks; too much vitamin A, for instance, can be toxic. Educate yourself about the right herbs and vitamins for your condition.)

- Know that you may confront negative reactions from others. Some people may urge you to follow the latest "miracle" diet. Others may tease you about your "rabbit food." Offer support to yourself for your efforts to maintain a healthy diet.

Reducing Chemical Exposure

Chemicals are everywhere. They're in your food: most vegetables contain pesticides and almost all farm animals are pumped with growth hormones and antibiotics. You breathe carbon monoxide, chromium, sulfur dioxide, and benzene during your morning walk. Indoors, you're exposed to even higher levels of chemicals, including formaldehyde in plywood and nitrogen dioxide from gas ranges (Harte et al. 1991). At work, pesticides are probably sprayed regularly in your office without your awareness. To completely rid your life of chemical exposure would literally mean packing up and moving to a hermetically sealed dome in the mountains.

While you can't eliminate toxins, there are ways to minimize your exposure to chemicals. If you are a person with chemical sensitivities, autoimmune problems, or asthma, reducing chemical risk is essential. Even if you don't have these types of hidden disabilities, your health may still be improved by staying away from chemicals whenever possible.

Where to start? First, do a careful walk-through of your home. Start in the bathroom. Read the ingredients on every product. If your shampoo or conditioner contains unpronounceable ingredients that read like a chemistry text, you may want to replace those products with something more natural. The same advice pertains to soaps, toothpaste, moisture lotion, deodorants, shaving cream, and makeup. Also, read the labels of cleaners and air fresheners. Some of these even have warning labels about product disposal and use with adequate ventilation. This means they contain risky chemicals.

Once you're done in the bathroom, review the products in the kitchen and laundry room. Check out the ingredients of detergent, fabric softener, carpet cleaners, and pesticides. All of these products pose some risk to you, especially if you're hypersensitive. While their use is widespread and socially acceptable, many experts believe that continual exposure to chemicals is dangerous.

Reconsider the use of these products. There are nonchemical alternatives with few or no artificial ingredients. (Yet, be forewarned: Some products advertise themselves as "natural" but have chemicals, such as fragrances or preservatives, in them. Read the ingredients labels carefully.) In fact, you can purchase all-natural products for almost every function in your household, from soaps to toilet bowl cleansers. Your local health food store is a valuable source of nontoxic household products. There are also mail order catalogues (see appendix D).

Here are some other ideas for reducing your exposure to toxins:

- Whenever possible, don't dry-clean your clothes. If you must, remove them from the plastic bag and air them outside for several hours before wearing.

- Avoid pumping your own gasoline. In some states, such as California, a gas station attendant must pump your gas if you have a disabled placard. Or you can ask a friend to do it for you.

- Be careful when installing new carpets. The fumes can exacerbate your symptoms if you're chemically sensitive. Ditto for painting or remodeling your house; even having your rugs shampooed releases chemicals into the air. Consider leaving the house for several days if you have work done.

- Avoid using pesticides. Research nontoxic forms of pest control.

- If you're moving, consider buying or renting an older home rather than a new one, due to the multitude of chemicals expelled by new carpeting, paint, floorboards, etc.

- Be aware of chemicals used at work. If you can, find out when projects such as painting and fumigating are scheduled; see if you can limit your time at the office on those days.

- Reduce exposure to electromagnetic frequencies (EMFs), commonly found in telephone poles and electrical devices like televisions and microwaves. Avoid having a TV in your bedroom, and place your clock radio away from your bed. If you're curious about the level of EMFs in your home, your local electrical utility company may be able to come to your home and measure them.

- Use glass containers in the microwave rather than plastic ones, as chemicals from the plastic can leak into food.

- Purchase several house plants, which are natural sources of oxygen; some plants can even remove gases such as formaldehyde (aloe veras), carbon monoxide (spider plants), and benzene (chrysanthemums) (Harte et al. 1991).

Mending Your Spirit

I used to be an upbeat and carefree person. But developing breast cancer changed me—and not necessarily for the better. I hear all the talk about how cancer is some wonderful opportunity. But, to be honest, I feel like it's squelched who I am. I want me back.

—Arlene,
a forty-eight-year-old teacher

Spirit is defined as "the animating force within human beings; vivacity; vigor." When you develop a hidden disability, you, like Arlene, may feel drained of this life force. It's hard to remain vivacious when you're depressed or your body hurts. Sometimes it feels like your spirit is just another casualty in the brutal toll your illness has taken on your life.

Your hidden disability can take you to the "depth of winter," as Albert Camus phrased it in the passage that we chose to begin this book. This period of darkness is marked by considerable loss and confusion. Your life is turned upside down. Many aspects of your life that you've cherished— like stamina, physical appearance, and work—have changed radically. Your faith in life and/or your deity may have been shaken to the core. You look in the mirror and don't recognize yourself. You wonder: Who am I? What's happened to me?

This period can be a dark and lonely one. Friends don't understand why you're so devastated by your illness and pain. They try to cheer you up with words like, "It could be worse. At least you're not dying." But they may not understand that in some fundamental way, you are grieving. You may not be terminally ill, but your losses are considerable. Your old body and life have "died," and you're trying to adapt to your new set of circumstances. Like the tribes who initiate their young people into adulthood by sending them off alone to fend for themselves, you've been forced to undertake a warrior's journey. It's not one that you've chosen. But it is one that you can survive.

Like Camus, who found that "within me lay an invincible summer," you can find your way out of the dark woods and reclaim your life. It won't look the same as before. But your life can offer profound meaning and deep growth. While it may feel like you've lost your spirit, the life force still exists inside of you. Your sense of your own spirit may be shaky and precarious. But who you are inside—your value and worth—is much greater than any physical or psychiatric disability.

To heal from a hidden disability means rekindling your spirit by finding ways to nourish it. You may find great comfort in prayer or attending church. Or, conversely, you may reject organized religion. Meditation and eastern philosophy may sustain you. Or you may not be interested in these practices and beliefs. Only you can decide what's nurturing for your spirit.

In this section, we'll describe the mind states that foster your spirit like, for instance, courage and forgiveness. We'll also suggest actions that fortify your spirit, such as altruism and compassion. As you read through the suggestions, you may feel skeptical, thinking, "How can I feel compassionate when I'm so frustrated?" Rekindling your spirit shouldn't be another stick that you hit yourself with. There will be times when you don't feel compassionate or peaceful. Know that this is natural, and accept that you're not perfect. Yet making an effort to incorporate some nourishing practices can offset the negative and discouraging times.

Courage

When you picture a heroic person, you may envision someone saving a baby from a burning building. It's hard to imagine yourself as courageous. But it takes great courage to live with a hidden disability. It requires inner strength to fulfill your responsibilities when you're exhausted or in pain. It's brave to confront doubt and skepticism from others.

Even if you're not aware of it, you manifest courage every day. You may feel weak and unworthy. Perhaps you beat up on yourself for not being more like someone else you know who seems freed of self-pity and anger. But know that feeling sad or angry at times doesn't negate courage. Courage doesn't mean fearlessness but, rather, an acknowledgement of fear and a willingness to persevere.

Chogyam Trungpa, a renowned Buddhist teacher, wrote about the "sacred path of the warrior" (Trungpa 1984). A warrior isn't aggressive; instead a warrior sees his or her basic goodness in spite of flaws and mistakes. To become a warrior means accepting yourself and your life. You have this ability to be courageous and to confront the challenges and difficulties that have befallen you. The trick is to start seeing your bravery and not just your fear. Courage comes from the root word "cor," which means heart. The more you open your heart and accept your vulnerabilities, the more courageous you will feel. You will also feel more encouraged and hopeful.

Arlene, a breast cancer survivor, felt ashamed to be so afraid. She envied other people in her support group who described cancer as a "learning experience." Arlene just felt angry, shut down, and depressed. She was shocked one day when a close friend expressed admiration for her perseverance in the midst of great pain and anxiety. At first she brushed off the compliment. But then she started realizing how brave she really was to undergo cancer treatments. As she put it:

> I was thinking of myself as a wimp. But my friend's words made me think twice. I have to go to doctors all the time and go for tests. I have to deal with the uncertainty of the future. I guess it does take courage to endure all of this.

Like Arlene, you accomplish heroic acts. To help you recognize your courage, make a list of ways you persevere throughout the day (however small these actions may seem):

_____

_____

_____

There may be times, however, when you don't feel particularly courageous. Perhaps you're drinking or eating more than you should. You may devote too many hours to worrying about your health. These are times when you want to fortify your "warrior" side. Here's an exercise to help:

> Take a few moments to relax. Find a comfortable place to sit or lie down. Breathe deeply. Now, recall a time when you went through a difficult experience. Take a moment to recall the details. How did you get through it? Think about the traits that enabled you to cope. Remember that you still possess all of these characteristics. Even when you're frightened or angry, you have the qualities inside that can tackle difficult experiences. Say to yourself, "I've gotten through difficult times before. I've survived. I'm a warrior." Whenever you feel weak or frightened, repeat this phrase to yourself.

Altruism

It's almost inevitable to become self-absorbed when you live with a hidden disability. You hone in on every ache and pain. You recount your new symptoms to friends and family. You worry incessantly when you're flared up. While common, this preoccupation can hurt your spirits. Self-focus makes you restrict your view of the world. You see only pain, uncertainty, and aloneness. To nourish your spirit you need to broaden your perspective. An effective antidote to self-focus is altruism or community service.

There are countless ways to give of yourself. Even small acts are powerful. For instance, Arlene became absorbed with her body, even after the doctors pronounced her cancer treatment successful. She worried constantly about a cancer reoccurrence and had frequent nightmares. Her partner, Lucy, expressed concern that she was drowning in worry and losing perspective on her life. While Arlene initially dismissed Lucy's concerns, she eventually recognized that worrying was unproductive. She resolved to do "service" for others to move beyond her self-focus. While her recuperation from treatment prevented her from certain types of volunteer work, she realized that she could call shut-ins and elders from home. The calls brightened the days of the recipient and made Arlene feel useful again.

Volunteer work is one way to be giving. But being altruistic doesn't necessarily mean joining a local organization. You can resolve to listen more attentively to other people's concerns. Sending a card to a loved one going through a hard time, donating clothes or canned goods, offering to take in a vacationing neighbor's mail, or greeting people with a smile and a "hello" during walks are all simple but significant acts of service.

Being generous helps others and boosts your spirits. Even if you don't feel like giving, find ways to stretch yourself. Resolve to do a giving act each week, however small. To get you started, here's a worksheet:

My altruistic action this week will be: _____

The benefits to others are: _____

The benefits to me are: _____

Solitude

Being alone doesn't necessarily mean loneliness. Solitude allows you to calm your mind, relax, and slow down. Most spiritual leaders spend periods of their lives in quiet contemplation. Making the time for silence and solitude can reduce your stress. You'll have the opportunity to befriend yourself again. Amidst all the busyness of doctor's visits, work, and seeing friends, you can reserve some time for yourself.

Solitude doesn't only mean lounging around at home watching TV. It means setting some time aside to truly be with yourself. You can take this time at home or outdoors. You can experience solitude while doing some activity or just sitting quietly. Eating a meal alone while appreciating the textures and flavors can be relaxing. Reading a book, sewing, praying, or meditating are other examples of solitary activities that can promote calmness and well-being.

The idea of creating solitary time may make you uneasy. Perhaps you're spending too much time alone already. When you're by yourself you may become overwhelmed with anxious thoughts. If you're concerned, start slowly, with just ten minutes or so. If you find that any time spent alone is too distressing, put the idea on hold until you're feeling stronger.

Here's an exercise that can help:

> Choose a peaceful place to be, whether it's at home or in the park. Take a few moments and just sit and look around you. Notice the sounds you hear, whether it's the refrigerator whirring, birds singing, or children playing. If you find yourself distracted by negative thoughts or worries, return to the sights and sounds around you. Look around at the different colors and sights. Simply enjoy sitting quietly and being aware of yourself and your world.

Community

While time alone is essential and replenishing, so is time spent connecting with others. Developing a community of supportive and loving people can ease your physical and emotional symptoms. Social support may help you to recover quicker from flare-ups, increase feelings of contentment, and perhaps even lengthen your life. Yet it's important that friends and family be understanding and empathic. Having critical or skeptical people around you is disheartening. You need people who recognize and respect your hidden disability.

Perhaps you already have a strong community. If so, consider yourself fortunate. It's all too common for interpersonal ties to weaken when chronic illness, pain, or psychiatric disability strikes. Maybe your relationships have suffered because you've become withdrawn or self-focused. Or maybe you've discovered some "fair weather friends" who haven't stuck by you during the hard times.

If you feel the need for more social support, there are many ways to achieve this. But it means taking risks and reaching out to others. Know that some friendships will work while others won't. Try not to get overly discouraged. You can make a plan to connect with old friends or make new ones. Here's a worksheet to use:

This week I will try to meet new people by _____

_____

I will reconnect with an old friend by _____

_____

I will strengthen my friendship with a current friend by _____

_____

I will strengthen my ties with a family member by _____

_____

Kindness and Compassion

When the Dalai Lama, the spiritual leader of Tibet, is asked to describe his religion, he responds that his religion is kindness. There's great power in bringing compassion and kindness into the world. But when you're living with a hidden disability, it's a challenge to feel compassionate toward others. You may envy their good health. Perhaps you're frustrated when some people don't recognize your disability. Feeling despairing and in pain can get in the way of being kind to others.

Yet closing your heart to others will further isolate and depress you. The increased tension in your body may exacerbate physical symptoms. Cultivating compassion is healing to your body as well as to your spirit. Following are some suggestions for strengthening your compassionate side:

- Remember that other people have troubles and heartaches, too. While it may seem as though you're the only one suffering, disappointment is a part of the human condition. When you envy others' apparent good fortune, remember that no one in life escapes losses, crises, and pain. There's an ancient Buddhist story that illustrates this:

  A young mother came to the Buddha carrying the body of her dead baby. Distraught, she begged the Buddha to bring the baby back to life. The Buddha said he would do this if the woman returned to him with a mustard seed from the house of someone who had known no grief. The woman thanked the Buddha and set off for the town. In the first house she asked the elderly man inside if he'd known grief. The young mother's eyes filled with tears hearing of the man's calamities and misfortunes. She entered the next house, and asked a woman whether she'd suffered. Again, the young mother heard sad tales of pain and loss. In house and after house, the same scenario occurred. Finally, the mother realized what the Buddha was trying to teach her: that suffering and loss are part of the human condition. She returned to him and asked him to help her bury her child; she also became one of his most devoted followers.

- Practice self-compassion. It's difficult to be compassionate toward others while condemning yourself. Take a few moments each day to honor how hard you're trying.

- As the popular bumper sticker goes, "Practice random acts of kindness and senseless acts of beauty." There are a multitude of ways to be kinder, from opening the door for someone to offering your space on line. These acts make you feel good about yourself. Kindness begets kindness; the recipient may consequently be more considerate of others.

- Recall the kindness of others. While you probably remember in detail every hurtful comment and action, it's easy to overlook the small acts of generosity and affinity. While some people have made thoughtless remarks about your hidden disability, others have been helpful and considerate. Whenever you feel disappointed with others, recall the tender and loving moments.

- "Metta," or loving kindness, is a Theravada Buddhist practice for cultivating compassion toward others and yourself. It involves repeating certain phrases to yourself that promote feelings of good will. You first bring loving kindness toward yourself, then toward those you love, then toward people with whom you have aversion, and finally toward all beings. Note that metta is not a form of wishful thinking; you say the phrases to foster compassion in yourself. Follow these steps to get started in practicing metta.

  - Step One: Repeat these phrases: May I be free from suffering; may I experience my true nature; may I have good health and well-being; may I live in peace.

  - Step Two: Picture those whom you love and repeat these phrases: May those I love be free from suffering; may they experience their true nature; may they have good health and well-being; may they live in peace.

  - Step Three: Imagine those whom you dislike and repeat phrases (adapt accordingly).

  - Step Four: Imagine all beings in the world and repeat phrases.

Gratitude and Appreciation

When you're ill or in pain, you focus on your losses. You're painfully aware of how much you can't do. It's harder to appreciate what your life does offer you. Yet, feeling grateful encourages a survivor, rather than victim, stance. You see the blessings in your life, not just the curses.

Zach, a twenty-five-year-old man with an adrenal problem, felt embittered about his disability. While previously active and fit, becoming sedentary and taking cortisone medication made his weight balloon to 250 pounds. He was embarrassed to date or to see his old friends. Distraught and overwhelmed, Zach sought help through a support group, where he realized that he wasn't the only one struggling. He also returned to church. His minister helped him to see that his life offered rich rewards as well as difficulty. Buoyed by the love and support of others, Zach became more active and optimistic again.

It can be a significant challenge to practice gratitude. Your initial efforts may, indeed, feel false. When you're angry and depressed, appreciation doesn't come easily. Yet, through disciplining your mind to also notice your good fortune, you'll eventually shift your focus. While you'll still be aware of your tribulations, you'll also be grateful for your blessings.

It's also important to learn to appreciate yourself. You're probably an expert on how to criticize and judge yourself. You recall every mistake you've ever made, every embarrassing moment. You reproach yourself for developing a hidden disability. Yet how often do you take a moment to value your attributes?

The concept of appreciating yourself may be a foreign one. Perhaps you don't even know how to start. Here's a checklist to jump start the process. When you become self-critical, you can use this list to remind yourself of your merits. If you're particularly hard on yourself, imagine your best friend checking off your characteristics. Check off those traits that describe you:

_____ You're a nice person.

_____ You're giving.

_____ You consider other people's feelings.

_____ You have a good sense of humor.

_____ You're a hard worker.

_____ You try hard.

_____ You're considerate.

_____ You're good with your hands.

_____ You're smart.

_____ You like to try new things.

_____ You're a good cook.

_____ You're loving toward your children.

_____ You're loving toward others.

_____ You try to work on your bad habits.

_____ You're a good friend.

_____ You're polite.

Now, add any other traits you value about yourself: _____

_____

_____

Following are some other ways to cultivate gratitude and appreciation:

• Remind yourself of the good things in your life. Complete this sentence: I appreciate the following things about my life:

_____

_____

• Make a list of people who have been there for you during the tough times:

_____

_____

Spend a few minutes feeling grateful for their presence in your life.

• Buy thank-you cards. Send one out whenever someone has demonstrated kindness, no matter how small. For instance, if the nurse in your doctor's office goes out of his or her way for you, send him or her a card. Not only will it please the other person, but also it will help you focus on appreciation rather than on disappointment.

Finding Meaning in Suffering

Everything in life is manageable if your experience contains seeds of meaning, according to psychiatrist and holocaust survivor Viktor Frankl (Frankl 1992). Even though Frankl endured unimaginable cruelty in the death camps and lost his entire family to the Nazis, he survived and thrived because he found purpose: He counseled other prisoners, maintained suicide watches, and created a theory of meaning called logotherapy. (Frankl wrote a manuscript of his theory that was destroyed by the Nazis; he later rewrote it.) Likewise, scores of other people turn tragedy into determination, including the founder of Mothers Against Drunk Driving, who focused her efforts after her child was killed by a drunk driver.

It's a challenge to figure out the meaning behind your pain and illness. What's the purpose of chronic back pain or Tourette's syndrome? What good could possibly be served by your gastrointestinal problems? Yet logotherapists believe that life always has meaning and that you can eventually find purpose. The word "eventually" is important, because it may take time and patience to discover meaning.

For instance, Andrew, a forty-five-year-old attorney with heart problems, blamed himself for "causing" his pain. His physical discomfort was compounded by self-hatred. Andrew saw a therapist schooled in logotherapy who helped him find meaning in his illness. Andrew realized that he'd devoted his adult years to the pursuit of money and success. He relegated his wife and children to the back burner. His hidden disability forced him not only to cut his work hours but also to change his priorities in life. As Andrew put it:

> I've been working my butt off since I was twenty-four. I've made partner, and I've earned a lot of money. But in the process I've been a lousy husband and father. While my heart problems have been absolutely miserable, they've also been a wake-up call. I've learned that I can't take it with me. I won't live forever. I'm grateful that I haven't had a massive heart attack and that my wife hasn't left me. There's still time to get my life in balance.

Finding purpose in your life doesn't mean glossing over the hard times. It doesn't imply that you're "lucky" to be afflicted with a hidden disability. It does connote, however, that there's something to be learned from every life experience. Here are some suggestions on how to derive meaning from your experience:

- Recognize your choices: You can choose how to respond to your hidden disability. Andrew viewed his heart problems as an opportunity to preserve his health and his family life. Frankl writes, "Whenever one is confronted with an inescapable, unavoidable situation . . . what matters above all is the attitude we take toward suffering" (Frankl 1992).

- Find meaningful activities: Discover activities that give your life purpose. You don't have to necessarily join a volunteer organization. Simply perform daily activities to the best of your abilities. Mother Teresa wrote that what you do is less important than how you do it: "It's not how much we give, but how much love we put in the *doing*" (Mother Teresa 1990).

- Distance yourself from suffering: See your pain as part of the suffering inherent in being alive. Your discomfort helps you to understand universal truths about illness, death, and impermanence. Rather than believe, "I'm a failure because I have a hidden disability," you realize, "Because I'm a human being, I'm not perfect. Illness is a part of life."

- Focus on others: Seek meaning through giving to others. If you're absorbed in your hidden disability, you'll lose touch with other aspects of your life. Even listening to a friend in need can get you out of your head and broaden your perspective.

- Discover personal meaning in your hidden disability: You can find purpose and meaning in your hidden disability. But no one can determine this for you. While friends may urge you to view your hidden disability as "a gift," this description may not ring true for you. Only you can discover the teachings rooted in your life. Andrew confronted his workaholism and his neglect of his family. For you, developing a hidden disability may have a different meaning. It may point you toward changing your priorities, self-acceptance, or asserting your rights. Again, the meaning is your own.

Forgiveness

Forgiveness is a controversial concept. Some religions teach forgiveness while rejecting normal feelings of anger, hurt, and betrayal. Yet, if someone hurts and offends you, it's natural to be upset with them. Immediately forgiving a person can happen at the expense of your own feelings.

There may come a time, though, when forgiveness could free you. Holding on to grudges makes you bitter and cynical. You don't need to forget what the person did to you. It may be appropriate to cool or end the relationship. Yet forgiveness recognizes that both you and the other are only human. Mistakes happen.

You're not forgiving the actions; you're forgiving the actor. If a friend, for instance, says that she thinks your hidden disability is psychosomatic, you're entitled to feel insulted. You may need to stew for a while. When you forgive her, you're not condoning her remark. Instead, you're acknowledging that friends hurt each other sometimes. Her intention was to help, not hurt.

But what happens when someone intentionally tries to hurt you? How can you forgive cruelty? This is a personal decision. If you've been sexually abused, for instance, you may or may not choose to forgive the perpetuator. By forgiving the abuser, however, you never exonerate the abuse. Brutality and violence are never acceptable. However, if you choose to forgive the person, you acknowledge that he or she is flawed, and yet is still a human being. You free yourself of the burden of anger and hate.

While you may decide to forgive certain people, the most important person to forgive is yourself. It's not your fault that you've developed a hidden disability. You didn't maliciously cause yourself pain and hardship. While forgiving others is optional, it's essential to forgive yourself.

The following sections take you through a forgiveness exercise, based on the work of Stephen Levine (Levine 1997). They are meant to be done while you're alone, when you're in a calm and relaxed state of mind.

Step One: Forgiving Yourself

Imagine the reasons that you're angry at yourself. Then say these words:

- I forgive myself for making these mistakes.

- I didn't mean to cause myself pain and suffering.

- I see that I'm only human.

- I'm letting go of anger at myself.

- I forgive myself.

Step Two: Forgiving Others

Recall a person with whom you're angry. (It's generally best to start small. Forgiving someone who abused you, for instance, may take some time and possibly professional assistance. Start with a smaller hurt.) Then say these words to yourself:

- I forgive you for causing me pain and hurt.

- I forgive you for making mistakes.

- You really hurt me, but I know that you're human.

- I'm letting go of my anger and hurt.

- I forgive you.

Step Three: Asking for Forgiveness

You may have hurt and offended others as well. Perhaps you've been gruff and impatient because of being in pain. Recall a time when you upset someone. Imagine you're saying these words to the other person:

- Please forgive me.

- I didn't mean to hurt and anger you.

- I'm human and make mistakes.

- I'm so sorry for hurting you.

- Please forgive me.

Creativity

When you're creative, you reveal your unique attributes. Yet creativity can become stifled when you're stricken with a hidden disability. You may not feel like writing poetry or listening to music. Your emotional life feels muted; it's hard to experience the passion it takes to be creative.

For instance, Mara, a twenty-five-year-old aspiring playwright, became depressed after developing a repetitive strain injury from her job. Her dream of writing seemed dashed. Since her world had been centered on writing plays, she despaired of ever being happy.

After a period of grieving, Mara realized that there were other options for expressing her creative side. She took a dance class, which elevated her spirits and offered her a creative outlet. She also experimented with other ways of keeping her play-writing dream alive, such as dictating into a tape recorder and using a voice-activated software program.

You may be able to relate to Mara's story. It may be hard, if not impossible, to sew, dance, draw, bake, or play the piano. Not only does your physical health limit you, but also if you're depressed, your creative side becomes dormant. Yet finding ways to be creative can enhance your feelings of well-being. Following are a few ideas for rediscovering your passion:

- See if you can still pursue activities you enjoy—with adaptation. If you love painting for hours, reduce the time. If you relish knitting, explore whether special wrist braces may help. You may need to consult with a physical therapist.

- If you can't do your usual hobby, find an alternative way to be creative. While you may grieve your old pursuit, the new one offers opportunities for self-expression.

- If depression is getting in the way of being creative, try some of the exercises we suggest in chapter 2 for ameliorating depression. Seek professional help if depression is debilitating.

Ways to Express Creativity in Everyday Life

Being creative doesn't always mean writing a story or taking a class. There are numerous ways to manifest your creative side. Here are a few suggestions.

- Bake a cake, using innovative decorations.

- Take photographs.

- Send a homemade greeting card.

- Plant flowers.

- Sing.

- Find a new subject of interest and read as much as you can about it.

- Write a letter to the editor.

- Cook an esthetically pleasing meal to share with a friend.

- Make a collage of pictures you've cut out along with your own illustrations.

- Take up haiku—short, yet expressive, poems.

Faith

Faith is a highly individual matter. You may find solace and inspiration in being a devout, church-going Christian. Or Sufi dancing may inspire faith. Perhaps you have a notion of some form of Higher Power that's undefined. Then again, religion and faith may hold no interest for you.

While faith is personal, studies have shown that believing in some force outside yourself is healing. More than 130 studies have demonstrated that prayer can improve health and happiness. For instance, cardiac patients who labeled themselves as "religious" survived longer (Dossey 1993).

Mara, who has the repetitive strain injury, described her faith this way:

> I was raised Jewish but never practiced my faith. To tell you the truth, religion always had negative connotations for me. But when I developed this pain condition, I started feeling differently. My wrist would throb in the middle of the night and I'd pray for strength and courage. I'm not exactly sure who I was praying to. But just believing that there's something bigger than me made me feel better.

Perhaps you've also discovered or rediscovered your faith. Or maybe you've lost faith since developing your hidden disability. You wonder how your deity, or the universe itself, could permit you and others to suffer so much. Rabbi Harold Kushner offers this advice if your faith has been shaken up: God doesn't create problems. Instead, God is there for comfort and solace when you're lost and in despair (Kushner 1990).

Again, faith is private and individual. If it's an area of interest for you, there are many ways to cultivate faith. The most popular form is prayer. Over 90 percent of men and women pray (Dossey 1993). Practitioners of many Eastern religions, such as Buddhism, meditate. There are various types of meditation, including sitting still and experiencing the present moment, focusing on a word (a mantra) or an object, or chanting. Meditating and praying build faith while relaxing and centering your mind.

If you're interested in exploring different religions, consider attending services. You can also explore meditation groups and centers. Consider reading books about the various religions and spiritual beliefs. You can even extract what interests you from each religion and formulate your own perspective.

Reminders

- You're the same person you always were.
- Your life force still exists within you, even though it may be subdued.
- Making peace with your body fosters healing.
- Try to forgive your body for causing you suffering.
- Tune in to what works for your body.
- You manifest courage each day by living with chronic pain or illness.
- Practice self-compassion and self-forgiveness. It's not your fault that you're burdened by a health condition.

CHAPTER **10**

Managing Pain
and Flare-ups

The turning point for me was when I realized that it was possible to control my pain—not cure it, but live with it anyway. Then I started feeling good about my life again.

—Robin, a forty-three-year-old
woman with temporomandibular
joint syndrome (TMJ)

Pain is deeply personal. What flattens one person hardly affects another. This doesn't mean that if you're in severe pain, you're exaggerating. Your experience of pain is based on a number of factors, including your pain threshold, central nervous system functioning, genetic influences, and emotional responses. Even if you're more sensitive than others to pain, your pain is still real.

Pain devastates lives. It wears down your body and spirit. Persistent pain leads to depression, despair, even thoughts of suicide. You feel betrayed by your own body. You run to doctors, take medications, and deplete your savings on alternative treatments. Yet oftentimes the pain continues.

The pain of a hidden disability can cause additional suffering because you may not feel that your suffering is legitimate. Some people say you're overreacting. They wonder how a "little" neck pain can cause such heartache. In contrast, someone with an obvious disability often elicits real sympathy. When a woman using a cane slowly navigates a crosswalk, others recognize her disability and may even want to help.

In contrast, when you appear able-bodied and healthy but walk slowly across the street, motorists may make an obscene gesture or honk at you. You look perfectly normal, yet you're getting in their way. Friends may groan when you again have to cancel an appointment because your back hurts. Thus, your considerable physical suffering is compounded by others' negative reactions.

Perhaps you question your own pain. If your doctors are skeptical, it's especially hard to believe in yourself. You may perceive yourself as weak and inadequate to be pummeled by pain that can't be measured. Or perhaps your hidden disability doesn't cause significant pain but produces incapacitating fatigue, allergies, dizziness, or flu-like symptoms. Again, lab tests may not detect abnormalities. Friends suggest therapy. You wonder whether you're a hypochondriac.

It's important to remember that medical science is in its infancy in understanding chronic pain conditions and immune disorders. Doctors are experts at evaluating and fixing broken bones. But when pain is unremitting, they often don't know why. The symptoms of chronic fatigue syndrome, fibromyalgia, and multiple chemical sensitivities, for instance, confound doctors. While they may attribute your pain or flare-ups to stress, the truth is that they simply may not understand what's going on with you.

Having pain that confounds medical professionals makes you feel helpless. You go to almost any length to feel better. If your best efforts don't work, you feel even more demoralized and depressed. Yet, there is hope. Chronic pain and illness flare-ups can be managed through self-care. Notice that we use the word "managed," because the hidden disability may not disappear permanently. If you've been searching for months or even years for a cure, you may be wearing yourself out with an unachievable goal.

Pain and flare-ups may not be eradicated forever, but they can be controlled so that your life is restored. Again, if you start feeling better, this doesn't mean that your pain wasn't real to begin with. Just as pain can be worsened through an unhealthy lifestyle and negative emotions, it can be reduced through positive actions. You can exert some degree of control over your pain. This chapter will show you how.

We'll explain the many dimensions of chronic pain—the physical mechanisms involved plus emotional components. By understanding and managing your emotions, you can reduce physical symptoms. While our focus is on physical pain, the same advice applies to illness flare-ups: Your attitude and behavior have the potential to either increase or decrease your symptoms.

The Mechanics of Pain

Pain often starts with an injury, accident, or operation. You decide to plant a garden after a winter of being inactive. While lifting a heavy bag of potting soil, your back snaps and then goes into spasm. You yell, stumble into the house, and fall onto the floor.

Physiologically, your body responds quickly to the injury. Nerve endings transmit information to the brain that you've been hurt. This information manifests itself as pain. Pain is a warning signal that your body has been injured. Because you feel acute pain, you cease the activity. Once you've begun self-care, the healing process begins. By resting, using ice, and taking anti-inflammatories, your back starts feeling fine in a few days or weeks.

But sometimes the pain doesn't go away as fast as it should. Or perhaps it stops and then returns, or travels to a different spot. After about six months, your pain is labeled "chronic." While acute pain is sudden and excruciating, chronic pain is usually dull, nagging, aching, burning, and tingling. Though not as agonizing as acute pain, the unremitting nature of chronic pain wears you down over time.

Chronic pain has been described by one pain expert as "garbage in the brain" (Marcus and Arbeiter 1995). Unlike acute pain, it serves no useful purpose. For reasons that no one completely understands, your nerve endings are still transmitting pain sensations to your brain even after the injury has healed.

Illness Flare-ups

Your hidden disability might not only cause pain, but also it may produce all sorts of uncomfortable sensations, such as malaise, exhaustion, and general feelings of sickness. Chemical sensitivity sufferers may experience skin eruptions or even seizures when exposed to certain substances. A CFIDS patient may be so exhausted that he or she has to literally crawl to the bathroom. Again, all medical tests may show up negative. Even with an illness that can be confirmed through lab tests, such as multiple sclerosis or lupus, symptoms may suddenly begin and then remit for no apparent reason.

What all these illnesses have in common is the unpredictable course of the flare-ups. You may be watching your diet, getting enough sleep, and combating stress through meditation, and yet you're flared up anyway. Or you try to do a task that everyone else can do, like go food shopping, and you're laid up for a week.

Sometimes you can detect a link between a flare-up and some activity. Eating spicy food may precipitate a bout of irritable bowel syndrome. An argument with your lover can trigger a recurrence of asthma. But, at other times, you have no idea why your illness has worsened.

You wrack your brain in search of the reason for a flare-up. Or you flagellate yourself for eating that extra egg roll or doing the laundry. Learning to live with your hidden disability requires both recognizing triggers and accepting that sometimes there are no triggers. While you can't always control flare-ups, you can control your reaction to them.

We suggest three approaches. First, acknowledge your flare-up. Expending mental energy questioning whether you're exaggerating serves no purpose. Most people don't want to be sick. Recognize your flare-up as a real, though unwanted, intruder. Second, view your flare-up as a teacher. Is there anything you can learn from it? Do this objectively, carefully reviewing what happened prior to a flare-up without using this information to beat yourself up. Remember, you're just a human being. Everyone makes mistakes. And taking some risks may be necessary as you learn what your limits are.

Third, recognize that flare-ups can't always be predicted and are part of having a hidden disability. One month you may feel fine after cleaning the bathroom. The next time, you're sick for days. Practice letting go, by realizing that you can only control so much about your health condition. Forgive yourself for being human.

Pain Medications

Pain medications can help or hinder. Medication can enable you to get through a flare-up, or it can prevent you from learning how to control pain on your own. The key is to strike a balance between over- and under-reliance on medications.

It's not uncommon for people with hidden disabilities to deny the extent of their pain and "tough it out." You may be embarrassed to take drugs for a problem that others don't recognize as real. Or, on the opposite end of the spectrum, you may be popping a pill at the first sign of discomfort. You don't want others to know that you're in pain, so you try to vanquish it. You end up dependent on forces outside yourself to reduce your pain.

Although you should consult your primary physician to help you use pain medications wisely, we suggest the following:

- Exercise caution in using narcotics, such as Vicodin or Percodan. These are powerful drugs that are physically addictive with long-term use. Doctors prescribe them for acute, temporary pain.

- For chronic pain, doctors generally recommend medications like NSAIDs (nonsteroidal anti-inflammatories, such as ibuprofen); acetaminophen; tricyclic antidepressants, such as Elavil; or muscle relaxants, such as Flexeril. However, be forewarned that even over-the-counter medication has potential side effects. Long-term use of acetaminophen (e.g., Tylenol) can produce liver damage. Ibuprofen (e.g., Advil) can cause ulcers and other stomach problems.

- Before taking any medication, research the pros and cons. Purchase a book on prescription medications or do a search on the Internet. Know the potential side effects. Don't be shy about asking your doctor questions. Pharmacists are also excellent sources of information.

- Don't be ashamed to use pain medications when you need it. Taking medications is not a sign of weakness or failure. If you have a debilitating headache that won't respond to relaxation techniques, taking an aspirin may be a loving act. At the same time, it may be wise to avoid relying exclusively on medication to manage pain.

The Psychology of Pain

Pain isn't just a physical experience; it's an emotional one as well. And your emotional and physical perceptions go hand in hand. How you view your pain can affect how severe it is. And the severity and chronicity of your pain will undoubtedly influence how intensely you experience it.

As an example of the interlinking of mind/body states, take Robin, a forty-three-year-old divorced teacher and mother of two. Robin was healthy and active until she developed TMJ (temporomandibular joint syndrome), which caused excruciating head and jaw pain, tinnitus (ringing in the ears), and dizziness. Five thousand dollars worth of dental treatments only made the pain worse.

Because of the unpredictable bouts of pain, Robin became tense, nervous, and angry. The tension made her tighten her muscles, producing more pain. She was stuck in a vicious pain cycle and was feeling increasingly depressed. After a year of agony, even the slightest ache threw her into despair.

While Robin's physical symptoms were difficult, her psychological state was even more debilitating. She worried incessantly about whether she was traumatizing her children. She regretted that she'd left her husband several years earlier, as she fantasized that he would have taken care of her. Since many of her friends and co-workers minimized her suffering, she ridiculed herself for being so distraught over, as she puts it, "a little jaw pain."

In desperation, Robin joined a pain management group. By meeting other people who understood her frustration, she gradually stopped being so hard on herself. She also learned many valuable techniques for reducing pain. While her symptoms didn't disappear, they did diminish. Robin also started seeing a therapist. By exploring her past, she learned the origins of her excessive fear and guilt. Armed with new insights, Robin felt more control over her life.

Robin's experience illustrates the crucial role of emotions in exacerbating chronic pain. You might find it helpful to investigate how your psychological state may contribute to your flare-ups. In the next section, we'll guide you in how to understand and control your emotional reaction to pain.

The psychological aspect of pain has three primary components. The first involves your personal history of pain. This includes the messages conveyed to you about illness, as well as your personal experiences of pain. The second component is your vulnerability to pain, which is both genetically predetermined and impacted by trauma. Negative beliefs form the third facet of the psychology of pain. Thoughts that are punitive and self-critical make any pain feel unbearable. What you tell yourself about your pain can cause endless suffering.

Your Personal History of Pain

Your perceptions of illness and pain took root in your upbringing. Messages about illness were transmitted to you both overtly and subtly. If you learned how to tolerate pain, you're likely coping reasonably well. If, instead, you inferred that pain was a sign of weakness or imperfection, then you may feel like a failure for having a hidden disability.

Robin, an only child, grew up with a mother who was chronically ill with severe migraines. Most of the time, her mother was bedridden with excruciating pain. When her mother felt better, she desperately searched for a medicine or treatment to ease her migraines.

Robin found her mother's illness hard to bear. Robin felt angry at her mother for so frequently being sick. Then she felt guilty for being angry. She sometimes wondered whether her mother was exaggerating her pain for attention. Since Robin's father sought solace through work, Robin spent long days alone in her room.

In therapy, Robin learned that she had unknowingly developed the following beliefs:

- Illness traumatizes family members.

- Illness causes family members to feel abandoned and alone.

- When you're sick, you must search outside yourself for a cure.

Given these beliefs about illness, it's no wonder that developing TMJ provoked massive anxiety. She was sure that catastrophe was on the horizon. When she'd get a headache, she feared she was getting migraines like her mother. She had the irrational thought that she was being punished for disbelieving her mother's pain. Robin assumed that she'd destroy her children's lives. She searched in vain for a "rescuer," who would cure her and save her family from ruin.

Robin's worries turned into full-blown panic attacks before she sought help through a support group and therapy. She realized that her illness was unleashing painful and long-hidden memories of her mother's chronic illness. The hidden nature of her disability made it hard to accept. As a child she disparaged her mother's suffering. Although this was a typical reaction for a child, Robin still felt intense guilt for doing so.

Now, as an adult, Robin was disparaging her own pain. She assumed that others, especially her children, would ridicule her as well. Robin needed to develop some compassion for the frightened and lonely child that she once was. By doing this, she could be kinder to the adult she was who had developed a hidden disability.

If you, like Robin, grew up with ailing parents or siblings, these memories may be complicating your current health problems. Even if you didn't face a health crisis in your family, it is still important to understand how you learned to perceive pain and illness. Answer the following questions:

What is a significant memory of illness or pain in your family? _____

_____

_____

How did you react at the time? _____

_____

How did others react? _____

_____

How did people respond to the sick person? _____

_____

What are some of the lessons you learned from this experience? _____

_____

_____

How can you revise these messages to be more positive? _____

_____

_____

Personal Experiences of Pain

When you were ill as a child, adults responded to you in certain ways. Perhaps your parents were doting and loving. Or maybe they were overwrought when you were ill. They may have been rigid and indifferent, forcing you to go to school when sick. These reactions impact how you face your hidden disability today.

Robin was a generally healthy child, but she was prone to colds and viruses. Whenever she would so much as sniffle, her mother would become fearful and take her to the doctor. Her mother continually feared that a cold would turn into pneumonia. Eventually, Robin became anxious whenever she felt sick. In college, she would race over to the infirmary if she felt ill. The nurse would need to reassure her that she was okay.

In therapy, Robin realized that she, like her mother, had developed excessive worries about illness. Her catastrophic thoughts about illness were rooted in the past, not the present, reality. Robin observed that she was generally a healthy person and had never even contracted the dreaded pneumonia. By seeing the origins of her anxiety, she learned to view her TMJ more realistically, thereby controlling her panic.

You, too, may have had personal experiences with pain that are clouding your perceptions of your hidden disability. By seeing the impact of the past, you can view the present more objectively. Answer these questions:

Recall a significant memory of being injured, ill, or in pain. _____

_____

How did others react? _____

_____

How did you react? _____

_____

What did you learn from this incident about pain or illness? _____

_____

How do you now want to view illness and pain? _____

_____

As a little child in pain, you may have felt nurtured—or abandoned. Being ill may have gotten you in touch with your personal power. Or, like Robin, you may have felt anxious and lonely. How you felt then will likely affect how you view your disability now.

While you can't undo the past, you can change how you relate to yourself now. Are you talking to yourself with kindness or hatred? Are you doubting your pain or believing in yourself? Regardless of your past experience, you can still learn to become the accepting "parent" that you longed for as a child.

The Culture of Pain

As a child, you were influenced by your family as well as the culture at large. You received directives early on about pain—how to avoid it, what it means if you get sick, how to deal with people in pain. These messages may have soothed you or agitated you.

Robin was raised in a Jewish family where many family members perished in the Holocaust. She recalled as a young child how her mother told her that to be Jewish means to suffer. Robin heard numerous accounts of how her family members suffered during the massacres of Jews in Russia and during World War II.

In therapy, she identified the negative statements she deduced from stories about her culture:

• Suffering is inevitable because I'm Jewish.

- There's nothing that I can do to avoid endless suffering.

- My TMJ is insignificant compared to the suffering of my people.

After reviewing her list, Robin recognized why she felt so helpless around her hidden disability. She had presumed that suffering was inevitable and that there was nothing she could do. She realized that this belief was irrational; there were many ways she could lessen both her emotional and physical pain. Robin also learned why she scorned herself for being overwhelmed by her TMJ. After all, given the "real" suffering her relatives endured, how could she complain about head pain? In therapy, she learned to accept her hidden disability as valid. Even though she hadn't lived through anything as tragic as the Holocaust, having TMJ was difficult and depressing at times. Chronic pain can sometimes feel like a prison.

Religion may also play an important role in how you perceive your health problem. If your religion preached that you should be stoic and ignore pain, you may be particularly self-critical. Maybe you were told that pain and suffering are punishments for your sins. But beliefs about pain can be challenged and changed. Here's a worksheet to help you understand the impact of culture and religion:

What messages did you receive from your religion (or lack of religion) about pain and illness? _____

_____

_____

What messages did you get from the media or culture at large about pain and illness? _____

_____

_____

How have these messages shaped your perceptions? _____

_____

_____

What are some positive beliefs that you would prefer to have about your hidden disability? _____

_____

_____

Vulnerability to Pain

The second component of the psychology of pain is your vulnerability to pain and illness. Some of this vulnerability is predetermined; qualities such as a high pain threshold may be genetic and inherited. However, life events will also directly impact your ability to withstand pain.

For instance, if you were sexually abused as a child, a hidden disability can evoke long-repressed feelings of helplessness and terror. Your body was exploited and used. You grew up feeling defective. By developing a hidden disability, you perceive your body as further damaged. Being ill and having to endure medical examinations can feel like further violations of your body. Abuse isn't the only precondition that can make your hidden disability feel traumatic; other difficult childhood experiences, such as loss of a parent or growing up with an alcoholic parent, may also reinforce fears that you're weak, inadequate, and powerless.

Here's a checklist that will help you to evaluate your vulnerability to pain.

Experiences during childhood:

_____ physical abuse

_____ sexual abuse or rape

_____ other traumatic childhood experience(s): _____

_____

_____ history of depression

_____ history of anxiety or panic

_____ family member with chemical dependency problem

_____ other family dysfunction: _____

_____ early loss (e.g., death of a parent or sibling)

_____ parents' continually discounting your needs and feelings

_____ difficult school experiences

_____ lack of support from your family

_____ other: _____

Current circumstances:

_____ people who discount your pain

_____ limited social support

_____ constant pain with almost no relief

_____ depression

_____ anxiety

_____ trauma related to your hidden disability (e.g., medical procedure)

_____ trauma not related to your hidden disability

_____ divorce or separation from partner

_____ death of loved one

_____ lifestyle problems (e.g., financial difficulties, unhappy living situation)

_____ other: _____

Review your responses. Any statements checked off in the "childhood" section set the stage for increased vulnerability to pain. Memories of these past experiences may be surfacing now that you're ill. Also, if your present life is stressful, any pain may feel intolerable.

If you are vulnerable to pain, it's especially important to learn to manage your pain. Here are some suggestions:

- First, recognize that you are more vulnerable to pain due to past and/or present conditions. Try not to blame yourself; the reasons may be out of your control.

- See what conditions in the past have made you more vulnerable. If you had some trauma to your body, you'll want to practice exercises focused on making friends with your body. (Psychotherapy or an abuse survivor support group may be warranted, too.) If there are current conditions that are increasing your vulnerability, see if you can change any of them. If your partner is unsupportive, let him or her know how this hurts you.

- Try this breathing exercise: When you experience pain, take a few deep breaths and say to yourself, "This is just pain. I can cope. The past is over. This pain has nothing to do with the past. Pain is a normal part of being human. It will come and go."

Negative Thoughts

The third component in the psychology of pain is negative thinking. Blasting yourself for having a hidden disability can intensify pain. For instance, take a moment and consider your automatic thoughts about your pain. Do you call yourself "stupid" or "weak" when you're flared up? Do you assume that the pain will never end? Do you blame others? Pessimistic beliefs may increase your pain. For instance, you arrive home from shopping and your back hurts. You think, "I shopped for too long! What an idiot I am!" These gloomy thoughts make you tense, and the tension produces more pain. You're caught in a vicious cycle that erodes self-esteem, confidence, and well-being.

The first step is to become aware of your harsh and dismissive thoughts. Ironically, you may be saying more hateful things to yourself than you'd ever utter to a friend. Here are some common negative thoughts. Check any that you're telling yourself:

_____ I'm weak. I can't even handle a little pain (or illness flare-up).

_____ I'm helpless concerning this pain.

_____ This pain will never end.

_____ Having pain means something terrible will happen.

_____ Being in pain again proves that I'm inadequate.

_____ If I were truly strong, I could overcome this pain.

_____ I'm exaggerating as usual and making a mountain out of a molehill.

_____ Other people would deal with this pain better than me.

_____ This pain is a punishment for my mistakes and deficiencies.

_____ This pain is due to bad karma.

_____ I must be cursed to be in such pain.

_____ I'm a victim of circumstances.

_____ It's totally unfair that I'd end up in this pain.

_____ There's no hope for me.

_____ Other: _____

If you tell yourself any of the above statements, it's no wonder that any pain feels intolerable. When you feel twinges of pain, it reinforces that you're a deficient, unworthy person. There are two ways to rework negative thoughts:

1. Start viewing your pain objectively. It helps to write on an index card, "Pain is a neutral event. Pain is just an unpleasant sensation in my body. Everyone experiences pain." Whenever you notice a negative thought emerging, read the index card a few times.

2. Rework your negative statements. For instance, if you agreed with the thought, "This pain will never end," a revision could be, "Nothing stays forever. Pain comes and goes, increases and decreases."

Robin, for instance, agreed strongly with the thought, "I'm weak; I can't even handle a little pain." She created this new statement to replace her negative thought: "I'm a success. I've persevered through a painful divorce and now a hidden disability. I'm raising two kids as a single parent. I'm trying hard to be happy even though I have TMJ."

Here's a worksheet to revise your negative thoughts about your pain:

Negative thought: _____

_____

Revision: _____

_____

Techniques for Reducing Pain

By now, you've probably gained insight into how your childhood history may have increased your vulnerability to pain. You've determined how current stresses lower your pain threshold even more. You've recognized the negative thinking that only makes your pain feel more intolerable.

You're now ready to try some methods that will enable you to cope more skillfully with your pain. These exercises take persistence and practice. We suggest doing at least one daily for a week or two to see if it helps. Experiment and see what works for you. You can also adapt any exercise to better meet your particular situation.

Method One: Reworking Past Experience with Pain

Is your current pain influenced by a difficult childhood experience? If so, try reworking this painful event and the negative messages that you still carry. (Note: If you find this exercise upsetting, immediately stop. You may need to do it only with the help of a trained professional.)

First, take a few moments to relax in a chair or on the floor. Breathe, and consciously relax your body. Then, recall an experience you had as a child ill or in pain. Take a couple of minutes to imagine what took place: where you were, what was happening, how you and others reacted. Notice how you were feeling. Recall other aspects of the experience: what the room looked like around you, what you were wearing, and any other details that you can recall.

Now, create a different scene: picture yourself in the same situation. But imagine how you would have liked people to respond. What would your parent say? What would a sibling be doing? How would you be feeling? What else would be occurring? Take a few moments to visualize this new and happier scene.

After you've finished, remember this scene, and know that you can return to it whenever you like. While you can't undo the past, you can create new realities for yourself. You can begin treating yourself in more loving and compassionate ways. You can also choose to have people around you who are caring and supportive.

Method Two: Rewriting Your Pain Script

Without realizing it, you've created a script in your mind detailing your hidden disability. Part of Robin's script went like this:

> My pain shows that I can't deal with life. I created this pain because I'm such a stressed out person. Now I'm making a big deal over a minor problem. People have cancer; they're the real heroes. Maybe my friends are right: I might be imagining the whole thing!

This script was causing Robin enormous misery. She rewrote this scenario to be kinder and more accurate:

> Having TMJ doesn't mean that I'm a failure at life. A lot of people have pain. And even if it's not cancer, the pain is real. I need to be more accepting of myself and try to relax.

Here's a worksheet to revise your own pain script:

This is my current script: _____

_____

_____

This is my revised script: _____

_____

_____

Method Three: A Pain or Flare-up Inventory

When you're in pain or ill, you may fear that you'll never feel better. Even when friends reassure you that your pain always fades, you're skeptical. Yet it's essential to see that pain comes and goes. While it can be intense and overwhelming at times, the sensations of pain are ever changing. A pain or illness inventory can help to convince you that your pain level varies and that you have more control than you think.

Or perhaps you have the opposite problem: You minimize or deny your pain. Since your disability is hidden, you may not feel entitled to have pain and flare-ups. Maybe people close to you diminish your suffering. Yet, by ignoring pain, your flare-up may increase in intensity. A pain inventory can warn you of the signals of a relapse.

Use a small notebook to write down your daily experience of pain. Record the information below four times a day, for example, when you wake up, at noon, around dinner time, and before bed. Here's a suggested format:

No pain/No stress   Severe pain/Severe stress

0   1   2   3   4   5   6   7   8   9   10

Time _____

Rate your pain (scale of 0–10): _____

Describe your pain: _____

Any triggers? _____

Rate your stress level (0–10): _____

What are you saying to yourself that is unsupportive or critical? _____

_____

What is a positive statement you can make about your pain? _____

_____

What can you learn from this incident of pain? _____

_____

One of Robin's entries looked like this:

Time: 8 A.M.

Rate your pain: 7

Describe your pain: pounding headache, especially around my temples

Any trigger? I slept poorly.

Rate your stress level: 8

What are you saying to yourself that is unsupportive or critical? That I'm going to be in pain all day.

What is a positive statement you can make about your pain?: I don't know this for a fact.

What can you learn from this incident of pain? I shouldn't have watched the news before I went to sleep. It got me all keyed up. Tonight I'll listen to my relaxation tape instead.

Method Four: Relaxation Training

Many people walk around tense and stressed out. Granted, there are inconveniences and irritations throughout the day: traffic jams, arguments, bills to pay. Having a hidden disability that causes pain while confounding doctors can make you even more nervous and restless.

Deep relaxation can be healing to your body and spirit. By relaxing, your muscles loosen and your mind calms down. Relaxation is something you may have to relearn. You've had many years of developing unhelpful habits such as clenching your jaw and tightening your neck. To release these habits, you'll need to decondition from your tendencies to tighten and stiffen. It's certainly possible to become more relaxed, but it takes patience and practice.

Here's a relaxation exercise to try. While doing the exercise, find a quiet and comfortable place to either sit or lie down. You can tape the exercise (remember to read it slowly) and then play it back. Or you can have a friend read it to you.

Begin by focusing on your breathing. Take a slow, deep breath. Breathe in, and then slowly breathe out. As you breathe in, imagine yourself bringing in healthy, healing energy. On your out-breath, picture yourself breathing out negative, unhealthy energy. Take another minute to just enjoy deep breathing.

Now, start with the top of your body and relax your head. Focus on your scalp and consciously relax. Move to your face—your eyes, nose, mouth, ears—and feel each part of your face and let the tension go. Now focus on your neck and shoulders. Imagine the tightness and tension melting away. Notice your back, and let any tightness go. Continue moving down your body to your chest. Breathe in healthy air and empty your lungs of toxic air. Move to your stomach, and relax your muscles. Relax your arms by beginning with the shoulder blades, then move down to your biceps, elbows, hands, and fingers. Let the tension go. Continue downward to your genitals, and relax this area. Relax your buttocks. Then imagine your thighs, knees, and calves, and let the tightness go. Relax the back of your legs as well. Move downward to your feet and consciously relax them. Take a minute and just relax and breathe. Notice if there are any areas of tension. Return to these areas and relax them. Enjoy the feeling of relaxation.

Variation

An alternative relaxation exercise is to consciously tighten and then relax each part of your body. For instance, tense up your neck muscles for three seconds, and then relax the muscles, letting your neck go limp. Continue to do this from head to toe.

Method Five: Autogenics

With autogenics, you reduce tension and produce feelings of well-being by bringing warmth to muscle groups. First, find a comfortable position and take a few moments to breathe. Then focus on different parts of your body, repeating these phrases: "My left arm is heavy. My left arm is heavy and warm. My left arm is letting go." Then move onto your right arm: "My right arm is heavy. My right arm is heavy and warm. My right arm is letting go." Continue to repeat these phrases from head to toe.

Method Six: Reducing Pain Sensations

Select one of the relaxation techniques just described. Allow your body to relax deeply. Then try one of the following pain reduction exercises. It's helpful to rate your pain prior to doing the exercise and then again right afterward.

- Imagine your pain on a movie screen in front of you. Now allow the screen to gradually move farther and farther away from you until you can barely see it.

- Picture your pain as having volume controls. Slowly lower the volume of your pain.

- Bring your attention to the part of your body that hurts. After a minute, look around the room and find another object to focus on. Concentrate on this object for several minutes. When your mind wanders, bring it back to the object.

- With your eyes closed, focus on the part of your body that hurts. Then scan your body from head to toe and focus on the parts of your body that don't hurt.

- Notice the part(s) of your body that hurts. Say to yourself, "It's just a sensation. There's nothing to be scared of. This sensation will come and eventually it will go."

Method Seven: Imagery

Guided imagery is an effective tool for alleviating pain and distress. Have a friend read you this script or make a tape yourself. This first imagery involves changing your conception of pain to a healing image. You can also substitute one of the other variations mentioned directly after the exercise.

Find a comfortable position and take a few minutes to breathe. Next, imagine walking down a staircase (or standing in an elevator), and each time you descend a step (or floor), you become more relaxed. Imagine yourself on step five, and relax. Step four, feeling more relaxed. Three, let the stress melt away. Two, feeling extremely relaxed. And one, feeling calm and relaxed from head to toe. Take a moment to breathe, and if any part of your body still holds stress, just let the tension go.

Imagine yourself in a lovely place; this can be a spot that you've visited before, or an imaginary place. Take a moment and visualize yourself in this beautiful locale. Experience what it's like to be there, all the sights and sounds. Imagine yourself just relaxing and enjoying yourself. Now, create an image that symbolizes your pain, for instance, a burning sun, the thorns of a rose, or a knife. Then imagine the sun cooling down or the flower losing its thorns or the knife's edge softening. Take a few moments and let the revised, healing image replace the original pain symbol.

Although you'll be leaving your special place soon, spend another minute just savoring what it's like to be there. Remember that you can recreate this scene in your mind whenever you need to. As your consciousness begins to return to the room you're in, picture yourself climbing the stairs (or going up the elevator). Step one, you're feeling more alert; two, you're aware of the sensations in your body; three, feeling more awake; four, noticing what it's like to be in the room; five, fully awake and alert.

• Variation 1: Imagine a being who represents healing for you; this can be a person, an animal, or a spiritual guide. Take a minute to visualize this being, and experience what it's like to be with this being. Picture yourself asking this being for comfort and for healing energy. Just experience how calming it feels to be in this being's presence.

• Variation 2: While you're in your special place, you find a scrapbook. You open it up and see that each page describes a challenge you've been able to meet in your life. You read about your courage and fortitude in facing these difficult experiences. On the last page, you imagine your bravery in living each day with a hidden disability. As you close the book, you're determined to remember all the positive qualities that you possess.

Method Eight: Affirmations

Affirmations are positive statements that you make to yourself. They challenge automatic thoughts that are pessimistic and self-loathing. Here are a few suggestions, with space to write your own:

• I can handle this pain.

• I am much more than this pain.

• This pain, like everything else, will subside.

• I forgive myself for being in pain.

• Ups and downs are normal occurrences in life.

• Even if others doubt me, I know that my pain is real.

- I am strong enough to endure pain.

- Other affirmations: _____

  _____

  _____

Handling Flare-ups

Here are some tips for managing flare-ups of chronic pain and illness:

- Schedule more time for rest. You may need more time for naps and sleeping in.

- Reach out for help. Have a neighbor walk your dog, ask a friend to bring over a meal, and request that your partner do the laundry. While you may feel uncomfortable asking, remember that most people enjoy helping out.

- Set limits. Say "no" to requests that aren't essential.

- Limit contact with difficult and negative people, especially those who question your hidden disability.

- Change your answering machine message to say that you're feeling under the weather, and that you'll return phone calls when you're better.

- Minimize stress. Avoid watching the news or reading the paper. If possible, put problems on the back burner.

- Add pleasure. Rent a humorous video, ask a friend for a back rub, take a warm bath.

- Remind yourself that this flare-up will end.

- Be kind to yourself. Practice stopping negative and self-defeating thoughts.

- Distract yourself. Read a magazine, go for a short walk (if possible), or call a friend and talk about his or her life.

- Seek support from other people in similar situations. Call a friend from a support group, write to a pen pal, "chat" with someone on the Internet. Keep the conversation positive and optimistic.

- Consider noninvasive pain control methods, such as biofeedback.

Reminders

Everyone has his or her own pain threshold. Remember that regardless of what other people say, your pain is real.

You can lessen your pain. While pain medications may help at times, you'll also want to try diminishing pain through learning different types of techniques.

There's an emotional as well as physical dimension to chronic pain. Consider that some of your anxiety about your hidden disability may stem from childhood experiences.

By trying alternative pain control methods, you'll increase feelings of control over your hidden disability. But be patient; it takes practice to learn to decrease pain.

Chronic pain and illness flare-ups come and go. See if you can notice triggers, but don't blame yourself if you suffer a relapse. Flare-ups are part of having a hidden disability.

CHAPTER 11

Navigating the Health Care System

My first physician seemed really interested in me—at least at first. But once he couldn't figure out what was the matter with me, he lost interest; he even seemed annoyed to see me. I've seen a slew of doctors since, every specialist you can think of. Yet no one has a clear sense of why I'm sick. I rarely go to doctors anymore. It's not worth the bother.

—Megan, age thirty-one

Undiagnosed Illness

When you break your foot, your doctor knows just what to do. Armed with the latest medical technology, he or she springs into action, ordering X rays, casting your foot, and writing prescriptions for painkillers. When you return a month later, your doctor removes the cast and offers you ideas for exercising your foot.

But what happens when, months later, you return, still complaining of foot pain? At first, your doctor considers other possible diagnoses, from gout to tendinitis. When more medications, tests, and an evaluation by a specialist fail to uncover the answer, your upbeat doctor may become frustrated.

And when you arrive at his or her office a year after your original injury, you may face a doctor with an entirely different demeanor. Annoyed and skeptical, he or she now probes your stress level, wondering whether you're depressed or anxious. When you tell your doctor that your only stress is this damn foot pain, he or she seems unconvinced. Your doctor finally pronounces your pain psychosomatic, offering you a choice of Prozac or psychotherapy.

Now doubting whether your pain is real, you choose to see a therapist he or she recommends. With no training in chronic pain or illness, your new therapist inquires about your childhood. Several visits later, he or she proclaims that your pain is due to "old wounds" and that once you heal your "unfinished business," your foot pain will vanish.

Running out of money and patience, you decide to check out alternative medicine. The acupuncturist you see attributes your foot pain to "unresolved anger." The chiropractor recommends ten adjustments at fifty dollars a pop.

Thirteen months, thousands of dollars, and ten practitioners later, a friend sends you an article on myofascial pain syndrome, a chronic pain problem believed to originate in the nervous system that causes muscle pain that may migrate to other areas. You recall how your neck and shoulders also ache, which the practitioners have dismissed as unrelated. While you feel momentarily elated to finally have a probable diagnosis, you wonder how on earth not one single clinician considered this possibility.

If any part of this scenario sounds familiar, you're not alone. Countless people with hidden disabilities expend a considerable amount of time, money, and mental suffering in the pursuit of a diagnosis and a doctor who understands. It's not uncommon to hear of someone seeing a dozen doctors and spending his or her life savings in quest of an answer to his or her chronic pain or illness. Others receive contradictory diagnoses from different practitioners, so they have no idea who to believe.

While you're searching, you may be fortunate to find a doctor who is supportive, empathic, and committed to working with you as long as it takes. But you may confront other types of practitioners, whether it's a physician who says your pain is all in your head or a chiropractor who's rushed and impatient. Finding the right doctor who will stick by you even if progress is slow may feel like the proverbial needle in the haystack. And perhaps, like Megan, quoted at the beginning of this chapter, you've become so discouraged that you avoid going to doctors unless you absolutely must.

Ironically, while finding a good doctor, a diagnosis, and a treatment plan may feel elusive, you never needed health care as much as you do now. When you were well, you only occasionally visited your doctor for a flu or sprained ankle. Chances are that you were satisfied with both your care and your insurance plan. Now, however, you find yourself dependent on a system that often fails to meet the needs of people with chronic conditions.

Becoming ill can also make you feel emotionally regressed. You're frightened about your symptoms and uncomfortable feeling dependent on others. You hurt and you want someone to reassure you that you'll eventually feel better. Since your disability is hidden, you suffer from doubt and uncertainty. Having a competent and caring doctor, then, becomes all the more important.

While dealing with the health care system may be arduous, there are ways to feel more empowered. It is possible to find clinicians whom you trust. Part of the solution is realizing that it's your body and you're ultimately in charge of your care. You'll need to be the one to advocate for yourself and assert your rights. While this is challenging since you're ill, it's not impossible. In this chapter, we'll outline ways to work effectively with doctors and other health care professionals. We'll also explore what you may be doing unwittingly to undermine your health care. With a change in your attitude and new tools at your disposal, being a patient may not be so formidable or disheartening.

The Search for a Diagnosis

Perhaps you were fortunate and the first doctor you saw figured out what was wrong. But for many people, finding a definitive diagnosis can be a frustrating experience, fraught with misdiagnoses, contradictory diagnoses, dead ends, and wounding experiences with doctors.

John's a typical example of the circuitous and frustrating road to a diagnosis. An athlete, runner, and self-described workaholic, John excelled in his work as a computer programmer. After a three-week camping trip, John developed a flu that went away after two weeks. But the symptoms returned months later. His knees ached so much that walking was difficult and running was impossible.

His doctor ran numerous tests, all of which came back negative. John had X rays done of his achy knees, and these were also normal. Yet John's symptoms only worsened, until he had to go on state disability.

For ten months, John went from doctor to doctor. All were baffled by his symptoms. Finally his family physician told him after the sixth visit, "Look, John, let me level with you. I've got a waiting room full of people who really need me. If I could help you I would. But, frankly, at this point, you need a shrink more than me."

Feeling humiliated, John became withdrawn and depressed. He spent days in bed contemplating suicide. His appetite waned and he lost twenty pounds. Finally, concerned friends arranged for him to see a psychotherapist.

Fortunately, the therapist was well-versed in chronic illness and pain. When John told him his story, the therapist said, "I don't think depression has made you sick; I think that you're depressed because you don't feel well and no one believes you. But I do."

The therapist helped John find a doctor skilled in helping patients with mysterious, undiagnosed chronic health problems. The new doctor immediately thought of Lyme's disease as a possibility, especially since the symptoms began after a wilderness trip. Even though other doctors had dismissed Lyme's disease because the test was negative, this physician explained that there are many false negatives. Once he began John on high dosages of antibiotics, John's symptoms began abating.

If you encounter doctors who dismiss or disparage your symptoms, it's easy to lose self-confidence. Like John, you may become depressed. Yet it's vital to remember that, much of the time, if you believe something is wrong, it is. You have lived in your body for a long time. While your condition may be worsened or triggered by stress, you still may have a real physical problem.

People tend to put doctors on a pedestal, elevating them to an all-knowing status. Yet, doctors are fallible like everyone else. They make mistakes and become irritable and burned out. And while doctors are adept at solving acute problems, such as bronchitis and broken bones, medical science has a long way to go in understanding chronic pain. And doctors' knowledge of immune dysfunctions, which are on the rise, is also extremely limited. When the tests return negative, doctors are often stumped. But this doesn't mean that nothing is wrong with your body.

How, then, can you as a nonphysician figure out what's wrong when the doctors cannot? This, obviously, isn't an easy process, but the first step is believing in yourself. It's vital to remain confident even when others doubt your condition.

Liz is a good example of someone who persevered and maintained faith in herself. A forty-three-year-old architect, she slowly developed a variety of symptoms that her doctor said would vanish on their own—only they didn't. Her ears rang, she was dizzy when rising, and she was exhausted. She had recurrent vaginitis and athlete's foot. Liz consulted ear, allergy, and dermatology specialists. All attributed her symptoms to a combination of stress and the aging process.

Liz cut back her hours at work, meditated, took daily walks—and still her symptoms persisted. She developed new, puzzling skin problems, like eczema on her hands and seborrhea on her scalp.

Time and time again, Liz would return to her primary care physician, who seemed dismayed to see her. He read through the chart while she told him of her latest problems. He looked at his watch when she asked questions. Finally, he told her that he couldn't help her. He suggested she find another doctor with whom she'd be "more compatible."

Feeling angry and abandoned, Liz decided not to allow her doctor's "firing" her to undermine her self-confidence. She'd always been healthy and truly believed that something was wrong—it was just that no one knew what it was yet. She resolved to find a doctor who believed in her and would stick by her.

Liz joined a local support group of people with chronic illnesses and asked around about competent doctors. She heard of a physician who was known to help people when other doctors were stumped. He introduced her to the alternative diagnosis of candida—a diagnosis that most traditional doctors reject. The doctor put her on a special diet supplemented with vitamins and medication. Within a week, Liz was feeling better than she had in a year. Several months on the regimen eliminated many of her symptoms.

Believing in yourself and maintaining hope are vital ingredients in your healing. There are many others ways you can help yourself while you're navigating the health care system. The following sections provide some recommendations.

Navigating without a Diagnosis

The first step is to become educated. The days of depending on the kindly family physician with ample time to discuss and research your case are long gone. Since it's your body, you need to become an expert in how it works—and how it doesn't. Check out the Internet, where you can both do research and chat with others who have similar problems. Obtain some good health books through a book store or your library (see appendix C for recommended readings).

While as a layperson you can't diagnose yourself, you can use the information you've gathered to ask your doctor questions, request diagnostic tests, and try noninvasive self-treatment, such as vitamins or special diets (although be aware that any radical diet or overuse of vitamins can be risky to your heath). Also, showing your doctor that you're informed can engender his or her respect, as your doctor can then view you as a partner in managing your health care. If, instead your doctor is defensive, he or she may not be the right doctor for you.

If you're not satisfied with your doctor, find another one. Most insurance policies allow you to switch. You have a right to a doctor who respects and listens to you. As a person with a hidden disability, you have the right to a doctor who:

Bill of Rights for People with Hidden Disabilities

- is trustworthy

- takes your symptoms seriously

- understands the challenges of having a hidden disability

- acts respectfully

- answers questions thoroughly and honestly

- speaks to you in language you can understand

- refers you to specialists when appropriate

- orders diagnostic tests when needed

- looks at your symptoms as a whole and sees potential relatedness

- recognizes that stress and depression are by products, not necessarily causes, of many health problems

- allows you to have copies of your medical records

- returns your phone calls in a reasonable amount of time

Continued on next page

- respects your right to pursue alternative health care approaches

  You also have the right to an insurance plan that:
- responds to your questions and claims in a timely manner
- authorizes appropriate tests and procedures
- allows you to see specialists and seek second opinions

Of course, it's best to work out a problem directly with your doctor. But the bottom line is that if you're unhappy with his or her knowledge base or bedside manner, you should consider finding a new health care provider.

How do you know when it's time to switch doctors? Take the following quiz to see how your doctor rates:

1. Your doctor is generally on time for appointments (give or take twenty minutes). *yes   no*

2. You feel comfortable talking to your doctor. *yes   no*

3. Your doctor takes your concerns seriously. *yes   no*

4. He or she gives you enough time. *yes   no*

5. Your doctor is patient with you. *yes   no*

6. Your doctor is interested in your case. *yes   no*

7. He or she remembers you. *yes   no*

8. He or she seems to believe that your symptoms are real. *yes   no*

9. Your doctor is willing to refer you to specialists and order tests. *yes   no*

10. Your doctor is open to alternative treatments, such as herbs or acupuncture. *yes   no*

11. He or she answers your questions. *yes   no*

12. He or she doesn't push you into treatments or tests. *yes   no*

13. Your doctor calls you back within a reasonable amount of time. *yes   no*

14. He or she is knowledgeable about your problem and up on the latest research. *yes   no*

15. He or she is willing to prescribe appropriate medicine and doesn't under- or overmedicate. *yes   no*

16. Your doctor is available in cases of emergency (or has a backup). *yes   no*

17. He or she is comfortable with your bringing another person to appointments. *yes   no*

18. Your doctor or his or her staff informs you of test results in a timely manner. *yes   no*

19. Your doctor's office staff is pleasant and helpful. *yes   no*

20. If your doctor has associates, such as nurse practitioners, you feel comfortable with their skill and demeanor. *yes   no*

If you circled "yes" for all of these answers, congratulate yourself on finding an excellent doctor. If you circled "yes" for eighteen questions or more, you still may be generally satisfied. However, if you circled "yes" for seventeen questions or fewer, you may be less than satisfied, and you may decide to ask around for information about other doctors.

Here's another good way to access whether you and your doctor are a good match. Look at the list of twenty statements, and mark the five that are the most important to you. Does your doctor meet these five requirements? If so, then you may want to stick with him or her.

Make sure that your dissatisfaction has to do with your doctor and not your health insurance. Some managed care plans limit your access to certain specialists or tests. Also, if you go to a large managed care facility where you see a different doctor each time, or doctors are allowed only a few minutes with you, you might be frustrated. Consider switching plans if possible.

Another thing that can be helpful if you haven't had a conclusive or satisfactory diagnosis is to get a second (or third or fourth) opinion. If one doctor says you have a herniated disc and need surgery, consult another before contemplating an operation (unless it's an emergency). While doctors are often adverse to contradicting colleagues, ask the doctor, "Would you get this surgery if you were me?" or "What would you advise your loved one to do?" Ask for a copy of your doctor's consultation report to ensure that you understand what he or she recommends.

During this time, it is especially important to trust your gut. If your doctor says your headaches are stress related and your instincts doubt this, you may be right. Again, doctors are fallible and make some judgments based on cursory reviews of test results and statistics. Your body is unique, and what's true for others may not be for you. If you believe that something is wrong, find a doctor who is committed to finding out the answer in collaboration with you.

Realize that you may not get a diagnosis quickly. In some cases, problems take years to be diagnosed—or the cause is never found. Again, an elusive diagnosis doesn't automatically mean that your problem is psychosomatic. While your doctor may not know what's wrong with you, you still may be physically ill. Of course, it's much harder to believe in yourself when you have no diagnosis. You may wonder whether you're exaggerating or overreacting. However, the place to start is within yourself. Remember to trust your instincts about your symptoms regardless of what medical professionals say.

Confronting False Assumptions

One of the reasons why you may not trust yourself is because you hold false or misleading beliefs about medical professionals. Since society reinforces the myth that doctors are always right, you may have a hard time standing up for yourself. In order to free yourself from these assumptions, you first need to see which ones you believe. Take a few moments to answer these questions about your unconscious assumptions. "T" stands for true, "F" stands for false. Circle the response that best fits your beliefs:

1. A doctor should be able to cure you.   *T   F*

2. Doctor are experts and they know what's best.   *T   F*

3. You should always do what the doctor says.   *T   F*

4. It's disrespectful to question a doctor's authority.   *T   F*

5. It's wrong to get upset with your doctor.   *T   F*

6. Your doctor is doing you a favor by seeing you; you should be grateful.   *T   F*

7. If you go to enough doctors, one of them will find a cure.   *T   F*

8. If you don't heal, you're doing something wrong.   *T   F*

9. You shouldn't undertake any alternative treatment that your doctor disapproves of.   *T   F*

10. If your doctor says that your symptoms are all in your head, he or she must be right.   *T   F*

11. If your doctor is arrogant, this is a result of his or her superior knowledge and expertise.   *T   F*

If you circled "true" for any of these statements, then you may be unwittingly relinquishing your power to another. You want to believe that your doctor has all-knowing powers so you'll be cured. Yet by elevating your doctor to a higher level, you may be discounting your own inner wisdom.

Here are some examples of how to change false assumptions to alternative, empowering statements:

False Assumption: It's wrong to question my doctor's judgment.

Alternative Statement: I am the consumer, and I have a right to be in charge of my health care needs.

False Assumption: A doctor should be able to cure me.

Alternative Statement: My body is what is doing the healing. The doctor may or may not have the answer for me. I'm doing my best to care for my illness or pain.

False Assumption: If my doctor says my symptoms are all in my head, he or she must be right.

Alternative Statement: While my doctor is entitled to his or her opinion, I believe that my physical symptoms are real, even if I don't have a diagnosis.

As an exercise, write down a false belief about health care providers and then come up with your own alternative statement.

False Assumption: _____

_____

Alternative Statement: _____

_____

After you've determined which distorted beliefs you're maintaining, you can then become a more realistic consumer of medicine. While you may wish your doctor had all-knowing abilities, you need to see him or her as a mere mortal. While your doctor's advice may or may not help, it's your body that's doing the healing.

To realize that doctors don't hold all the answers can be scary. You may feel alone with your problems. When ill, you may regress to a childlike level where you hope for a parent figure to take care of you. Yet the truth is that you're ultimately responsible for yourself.

It can feel empowering to know that you hold the key to healing. Rather than looking outside for the answer, your own instincts guide the way. If you notice a certain diet helping, then this information is most important. By looking within and trusting your intuition, you'll take a giant step forward in your recovery.

Dealing with Challenging Situations

Once you've gotten in touch with your own authority and personal power, you are in a better position to confront difficult situations. As someone with a hidden disability, you attend more medical appointments than you have in the past.

Perhaps your doctors are genuinely concerned, caring, and affirming. Or, conversely, you may have to confront difficult situations, such as practitioners who disqualify your symptoms, are condescending, fail to refer you to specialists, or are outright hostile. This is especially harmful since you're dealing with all this at a time when you feel vulnerable, frightened, and dependent.

You may return from a doctor's visit feeling confused or frustrated. Perhaps the doctor spoke too fast, used overly technical language, or was vague when answering your questions. Maybe you became intimidated by his or her white coat and forgot to ask the questions you meant to ask. Or maybe your doctor was disqualifying, and you're now kicking yourself for not speaking up for yourself.

One way to deal with challenging situations is to come prepared. Sitting in a paper gown in a cold exam room is not the best place to think of a snappy comeback to an insensitive remark. Planning for doctor's visits in advance can increase the chances of a positive experience.

Some tips:

Write down symptoms and dates they started. Send for medical records and bring copies of these to appointments. When you arrive, hand the records to office staff so the doctor can read them prior to seeing you. Bring a friend with you if possible to help you remember what the doctor said and to ask questions you might not think of. Consider tape recording your visit, with your doctor's permission; you can replay the tape later to refresh your memory.

Yet, even when you're prepared, difficult situations may arise. The following sections describe some examples—with possible solutions.

"It's All in Your Head." Responding to the Skeptical Practitioner

You are presenting your very real symptoms to a nurse practitioner, yet he or she expresses doubt.

Nurse: So you've been feeling exhausted for two months. And you've had headaches almost every day. Have you been stressed out?

Patient: Before I got sick my life was going pretty well. I feel stressed out about being sick and tired all the time.

Nurse: I see on your medical history form that you've seen a therapist for two years. Are you depressed?

Patient: No, actually I've been in therapy to help with some career changes.

This conversation isn't going in a helpful direction. The nurse's questions are making you feel like a hypochondriac. If you don't say anything, you may leave feeling offended and disqualified. But if you get hostile, you'll alienate him or her, and this office has an excellent reputation. Here's one approach:

Patient: You seem like a very knowledgeable practitioner. As I mentioned to you, I'm having some physical problems and I don't know why. I'm counting on you to help me figure out what could be happening medically.

Nurse: Yes, but stress and depression can cause fatigue and headaches.

Patient: I'm willing to consider this possibility, but only after physical problems have been ruled out. Now let's focus on what medical problems could be causing my symptoms.

This approach is both respectful and determined. You're open to what he or she says, but you're determined to focus on medical, not psychiatric, possibilities.

"Have You Given Up on Me?" When Your Doctor Dismisses Your Symptoms

You've been seeing your doctor for several months. At first he or she was interested and sympathetic. But your doctor seems less than thrilled to see you for the fifth time. You bring in a list of new symptoms and tests you'd like ordered:

Patient: I've had two migraine attacks in the last two weeks. I've never had a migraine headache in my life.

Doctor: *(writing down notes)* Everyone gets a headache from time to time.

Patient: It wasn't just a headache—it was a migraine. And I've read that it can be significant to suddenly get migraines after age forty.

Doctor: I wouldn't worry about it.

Patient: And I'm cold all the time. I just can't warm up.

Doctor: *(walking out)* You're thin, so you probably get colder than other people. You'll be fine.

Patient: Doctor, please don't leave yet. I want to let you know that I appreciate all your help with my health problems. I'm sure it's hard that I come in here frequently with different symptoms. But you seem to be dismissing my concerns. Given that I've been sick for almost a year, these new symptoms may be significant. I need your help in figuring out the possibilities.

In this dialogue, you're letting your doctor know that you're concerned about your symptoms—and that he or she needs to be as well. You're doing so in an assertive, not aggressive, manner. Yet what happens if your doctor continues to dismiss you?

One option is to write your doctor a letter after the appointment (and after your anger has cooled down). Here's an example:

Dear Doctor _____:

After our appointment today, I wanted to write you with some concerns. When I first started seeing you for my digestive problems, you were very helpful. I really appreciated the time you took with me. But today I felt that you were minimizing my concerns. Your intention may have been to reassure me, but it had the effect of making me feel you weren't taking me seriously.

I had been feeling optimistic that together we'd figure out what's wrong with me and what might help. Now I wonder whether you're burned out on my case. I know that you're a very busy doctor, but I hope that you're still willing to work with me to figure out what's wrong. I look forward to hearing from you.

Sincerely,

(Your name)

The style of this letter is direct yet respectful. You're conveying that you need your doctor's help and that his or her expertise is essential. At the same time, you're clear that your doctor needs to pay more attention to your concerns.

"Why Are You Treating Me This Way?" Dealing with Hostility or Insensitivity

You've waited two months to see a top orthopedic surgeon. The opulent waiting room boasts a panoramic view of the city. An hour after your appointment time, you're escorted to the exam room, where you wait another twenty minutes in a cotton gown. The doctor enters and says, "How can I help you?"

Patient: I was in a car accident a year ago and I'm still having pain in my neck and shoulders. The pain travels down to my . . .

Doctor: I see that you already had an MRI done. (*Looking at the MRI.*) It looks fine to me.

Patient: Well, that may be true, but I'm in pain all the time. I can't do my usual work of graphic design, and I've had to . . .

Doctor: Well, look, you're forty-seven years old. You don't heal so quickly when you're middle-aged.

Patient: That may be the case, but still I have a burning sensation in my wrist and my fingers get numb and sometimes . . .

Doctor: I don't know what else I can tell you. You had an MRI, and it's perfectly normal. Look, you're no spring chicken anymore. At your age, everyone has some aches and pains. Get used to it!

At this point, you're either furious or beset with self-doubt. With either reaction, you're not getting what you set out for, which is this doctor's expertise. You might try the following approach:

Patient: Doctor, I know that you're very busy and your time is valuable. But I'm in pain, and it's taken me two months to see you. I'd like you to examine me and tell me the possible reasons for this pain.

Doctor: The MRI is negative! There's nothing wrong with you. Do you want me to make something up?

Patient: Doctor, I'm in pain, and I feel like you're mocking me. Are you willing to examine me and help me figure out what I can do about this pain?

When a practitioner is hostile, you need to confront him or her and redirect the conversation. However, if the doctor continues to be disparaging, you'll need to leave. Regardless of a practitioner's reputation or training, he or she has no right to be rude or hostile to you. You should consider writing a formal complaint letter to your insurance plan and requesting another consultation with a different doctor.

"I Can Treat You Myself." When Your Doctor Won't Refer You

In this age of managed care, doctors may be averse to referring you to specialists or to authorize tests since they often have to foot the bill (see explanation in later section regarding what your doctor's experiencing). Here's one way to address this problem.

Doctor: Looks like your thyroid test is negative. So we can rule out a thyroid problem.

Patient: But, Doctor, last time you said that all my symptoms pointed to an underactive thyroid.

Doctor: True, but this test has ruled that out.

Patient: I'd really like to consult with an endocrinologist. I hear that there's other specific thyroid tests that an endocrinologist can run.

Doctor: Like I said, the test was negative. We can run some more blood tests to rule out other problems.

Patient: I appreciate your knowledge and expertise. But in this case I'd like to see a specialist.

Doctor: Let's run a few more tests first.

Patient: Doctor, I'd like to see a specialist. When can you arrange this?

At this point, the doctor will either accommodate your request or refuse. You can continue to use this "broken record" technique by asserting your wishes again and again. If your doctor refuses, you can either write him or her a letter with a formal request or call your insurance company. If your doctor appears overly frugal about referrals, you may need to consider transferring to a different primary care physician.

"Let Me Worry About It." The Paternalistic Practitioner

When you were well, you appreciated your doctor's reassuring style. However, now that you have health problems, you find his or her false reassurances condescending. You want to play more of a role in making health care decisions, and you desire more information.

Patient: I see that one of my blood tests came back positive. What does this mean?

Doctor: Don't worry about it for now. First let's get all the tests results back, and then I'll interpret them for you.

Patient: But isn't this a possible sign of a serious immune problem?

Doctor: Don't worry yourself for nothing! When I finish doing all the testing, then I'll let you know my final diagnosis.

Patient: Doctor, I know that you deal with all types of patients. I'm sure that many people prefer to not know that much about their tests. However, I'm the type of person who wants to be kept as informed as possible. You don't need to protect me. Now, please explain the implications of this positive test result.

"Let's Do It Now." Dealing with Pushy Practitioners

Your knees have been hurting more than ever. It's taken ten days to get in to see your rheumatologist. He or she does a quick check and then says:

Doctor: Yeah, they're inflamed. Let's do a cortisone injection. You'll feel much better within days.

Patient: (*nervously*) A cortisone injection? Aren't there risks in that?

Doctor: Hardly any at all. I do them all the time. Do yourself a favor and you'll be thrilled with the results.

Patient: Uh, I don't know.

Doctor: Look, it's up to you. But I don't have all day. What do you want to do?

In this case, the doctor is pressuring you without providing adequate information about risks and side effects. Your instincts are saying "no," but you also want to feel better. What should you do?

The general rule is to trust your instincts. If you're feeling uncomfortable and unsure, then wait. Most procedures for nonemergencies can be delayed. See if your doctor can be clearer about the pros and cons. Once you have done some research and collected your thoughts, you can either go back for the injection or skip it. Say to your doctor, "I appreciate this option. But I need to think about it. Can you explain more about possible risks?"

"Don't Waste Your Money on Hocus Pocus." When Your Doctor is Close-Minded

After trying almost everything western medicine has to offer, you turn to alternative medicine to help with your back problems. Treatment by a Rolfer (a type of bodyworker) has significantly lessened the pain. When you see your doctor, you report your success.

Patient: I'm feeling much better since a few of these Rolfing treatments.

Doctor: Well, I'm glad you're feeling better. But I think that it's probably the medication I gave you last time.

Patient: Actually, I stopped taking the medication because it was giving me stomach trouble. I'm sure it's the Rolfing.

Doctor: (*chuckling*) Whatever you say. But I think it's probably a placebo effect more than anything else.

By now, you may be steaming because your doctor isn't taking you seriously. But since you generally value your doctor's knowledge, you don't want to alienate him or her. Here's a possible response:

Patient: Doctor, I hear what you're saying, that you don't believe in Rolfing. And you are, of course, entitled to your opinion. But I want to try some alternative approaches since just taking medication isn't a cure either. I hope that you'll be open to hearing about my experiences using alternative treatment.

You might also find your doctor to be skeptical, disparaging, or even outright hostile regarding alternative medicine. He or she may feel that if a treatment hasn't been studied using standard research techniques, it's of dubious value. Perhaps your doctor wants to save you the time and expense. Maybe your doctor feels threatened because he or she has little knowledge about the treatment.

There are many other doctors, however, who are curious about and interested in different treatments, even if they're unorthodox. See if your doctor is willing to be educated about your new approach; offer him or her some written information. If your doctor remains leery and his or her support is essential to you, consider finding another doctor.

Here are some other tips for working well with health care practitioners:

- Choose your battles. If your doctor is generally helpful but is having an off day, give him or her the benefit of the doubt. However, if there's a pattern emerging of disinterest or skepticism, you'll need to speak to your doctor about the problem.

- Connect with others who have a similar health problem. Network together and talk about highly regarded doctors and treatments worth trying.

- Be aware if you are being curt or abrupt with your doctor. The doctor/patient relationship is a partnership. Take responsibility for your own reaction, and, if you responded unfairly, apologize. (We'll talk more later in this chapter about possible versions of your doctor's experience.)

- Know when it's time to take a break from searching for a diagnosis or treatment. The pursuit is exhausting, time-consuming, and emotionally grueling. You may need to change your mind-set from focusing on finding a cure to enjoying your present life to the best of your ability. Remember that choosing to stop treatment is not admitting defeat. Instead, it's an act toward moving on and living fully in the present moment.

When Healers Hurt You

Turn on any television newsmagazine and you'll hear plenty of stories about patients who've been injured by health care professionals, some of whom are well-meaning, others who've been proven incompetent. Are these isolated incidents exploited by the media? Or can health care itself be hazardous to your health?

Medications, surgery, and injections can be miraculous; yet, they also have the ability to injure you, an effect called "iatrogenic," meaning damage resulting from medical science itself. All drugs have potential side effects. An operation that can cure one person can paralyze another. And traditional, Western medicine is not the only culprit of iatrogenic effects. Alternative medicine, such as acupuncture, chiropractic, naturopathy, and herbalogy, can also cause harm.

Here are some real-life examples:

- A woman with a back problem sees a massage therapist for thrice-weekly sessions. His technique is vigorous and painful. She's concerned but assumes that the harder the massage, the better. He ends up causing permanent muscle damage.

- A man with a chronic rectal pain problem sees an acupuncturist who suggests a "harmless" procedure involving removal of some tissue in his lower back. The man is wary, but defers to the acupuncturist, who has an excellent reputation. This excruciating procedure results in residual nerve pain.

- A woman with an undiagnosed problem with back pain sees a chiropractor who convinces her to come for aggressive adjustments five times a week. She wonders whether this is too much, but feels uncomfortable questioning his judgment. The treatments cause her disc to rupture, requiring emergency surgery.

- A woman with rosacea (a facial skin disease) sees a naturopath who recommends taking hydrochloric acid nutritional supplements several times a day. The woman trusts this highly recommended naturopath and takes the supplements without question. She develops a preulcerous condition.

While it can be frightening to read these stories, knowing the risks can enable you to become an educated consumer. Both traditional and alternative medicine can be tremendously helpful—but they also have the potential to hurt. As someone with a hidden disability, you are especially susceptible to risky treatments because you feel badly and desperately want to get better. Since your health problems are not always recognized by others, you're more likely to feel ashamed and self-doubting. A practitioner offering a quick fix or miracle cure can be very appealing.

What are some ways to protect yourself against iatrogenic effects? The keys are becoming informed, learning the pros and cons of each treatment, talking with others, asking questions, and not rushing into anything.

Here's some additional advice:

- Trust your instincts. Many of the people in the above examples felt uncomfortable with their practitioner's recommendations, but they ignored their instincts. They were intimidated by their clinicians' power and authority—and they wanted to feel better right away. They so much wanted to believe in the practitioner that they stopped believing in themselves.

- Take your time and don't rush into anything. Thoroughly research the potential problems versus the benefits. Then you can make your final decision, fully aware of the risks.

- Read about medications before taking them. Consider starting with a very low dose to see what kind of reaction you may have. Your local pharmacist is a valuable resource to answer questions about possible side effects. Make sure to discuss the potential side effects of combining medications. And remember that just because a medication is sold over the counter doesn't necessarily mean it's free of side effects.

- Look into the possible hazards of nutritional supplements, herbs, and vitamins. Taking a large number of vitamins and other supplements a day can produce side effects. Start slowly, and stop or reduce any vitamin that's causing problems.

- Educate yourself before undergoing any procedure or operation. Get a second opinion. Speak to others who have had the procedure and ask them about their experience, including complications. Call your state's regulatory medical board to find out whether your practitioner has had any complaints filed against him or her. Know all the risks before making a final decision.

Your Doctor's Experience

The patient/doctor relationship is a two-way street. To be successful, you need a clinician to support your viewpoints and to be responsive to your needs. At the same time, you also have a responsibility to the relationship. Without realizing it, you might be impeding the alliance by being too passive or, conversely, overly demanding. Understanding the pressures and limitations your doctor faces can help you to become more tolerant, thereby increasing the chances of a positive experience.

Most doctors choose their profession to help and to heal. They feel enormously gratified when a sick person becomes well and when an operation is successful. Doctors are trained to fix, cure, and vanquish pain. They depend on an armament of pills, procedures, and tests to help them restore health.

Yet, in some cases, patients don't get well. They don't die, either. Instead, problems become chronic. The same patients come back time and time again with the same symptoms or new, puzzling ones. And even with all their training and tools, the doctor can't figure out what's wrong.

Consider a typical day in the life of a primary care physician. The first patient he sees was treated a few months ago for pneumonia. After rest and antibiotics, the patient is back to her rigorous, vibrant self. The patient offers the doctor heartfelt thanks, and the doctor is delighted by the patient's rapid recovery.

The next patient is Patricia, a forty-five-year-old woman who's been sick for eighteen months. This is her tenth appointment with the doctor. Her symptoms are puzzling and mysterious: nausea and dizziness with exposure to chemicals, rashes, immense fatigue, and sinus infections.

The doctor groans silently at the prospect of seeing Patricia. He has already referred her to several specialists and run costly tests. Yet nothing has shown up.

Today, Patricia comes in with an article on multiple chemical sensitivities (MCS). In the doctor's eyes, Patricia is a middle-aged, childless woman with too much time on her hands and a hypochondriacal fixation on her body. The doctor tells her that it's time for her to see a psychiatrist.

From this doctor's point of view, Patricia is a difficult, frustrating, and expensive patient. She's never satisfied with her doctor's opinions, and this bruises his ego. She wants more testing and referrals to specialists, which her doctor resents because it comes out of his pocket. (Due to a common arrangement with her managed care company known as "capitation," the doctor receives a fixed fee to see Patricia, and costs for specialists and tests come out of this fee.) And she presents hypothetical diagnoses that in her doctor's mind are unscientific and far-fetched, like MCS.

While it may be easy to condemn such doctors, the reality is that they are human. When doctors can't help, they often become frustrated. When a patient costs more money than others, they may wish that the patient would go elsewhere. And there are added pressures: Many managed care plans penalize doctors for running too many tests. Some insurance companies require doctors to see patients for only ten minutes or so. Doctors also have to spend more time on the phone gaining approval for tests and specialists.

Practitioners have some legitimate gripes about patients who are disrespectful, unreasonable, or demanding. Without realizing it, you may be acting in ways that are undermining your health care or alienating your health care professional. If you are, it's essential that you recognize this and change your stance. A respectful, collaborative working relationship is vital for you to get your health care needs met. Also, feeling trust and faith in your doctor can have a reassuring and even healing effect on your mind and body.

Review the following scenarios and see whether you recognize yourself in any of them:

- You come braced for battle, with an angry, chip-on-the-shoulder attitude.

- You present your symptoms in a vague manner, bring no notes to help you, and are unsure of chronology and dates.

- You push for more pills, even though you have other prescriptions and your doctor expresses concern over your use of pain medications.

- You are extremely defensive when your doctor asks you whether you're depressed, immediately assuming he or she is doubting your symptoms.

- You inundate your doctor with long-winded accounts of every ache and pain.

- You don't tell your doctor everything, such as about having panic attacks, because you fear being labeled a hypochondriac.

- You ask too many questions without sensitivity to the time limits.

- You repeatedly act pleasant to your doctor but then register complaints behind his or her back.

- You're rude and pushy to office staff and assistants.

- You make unreasonable demands on office staff without sensitivity to their busyness.

- You demand that your doctor see you or call you immediately for non-emergency situations.

- You pressure your doctor for tests that he or she says are unnecessary or redundant.

- You expect your doctor to be your therapist and speak at length about your emotional concerns.

- You call your doctor after hours for nonemergencies.

- You don't follow your doctor's suggestions around healthy living, such as stopping smoking, reducing alcohol use, and eating better.

- You bring an aggressive friend with you who makes the doctor feel ambushed.

- You avoid going to the doctor until your problems are extreme, and then demand instant relief.

Do any of these sound familiar? If you're coming across as too demanding, this may be because you're frustrated by being ill for so long. It's hard to be mellow when you're in pain. And if you're defensive when your doctor asks about your emotional state, this may be because others in your life are questioning your physical symptoms. Or perhaps you're intimidated by the doctor and withhold information or resist his or her attempts to help you.

Your sense of anger, helplessness, and frustration may make you a difficult patient. If you're unwittingly contributing to problems with your doctor, find ways to restore the patient/doctor alliance. A trusting and supportive relationship with your doctor is vital when you have a hidden disability. Here are some suggestions:

- Recognize that your doctor is probably trying his or her best to help you. Your doctor also wants you to feel better. But your doctor is human, too. He or she has bad days and gets burnt out. And since your doctor isn't omniscient, his or her knowledge base is sometimes limited.

- Don't personalize your doctor's behavior. If your doctor is curt or impatient with you, consider that your doctor may have been up all night with his or her own children or had to see a patient at the hospital until late. If your doctor is reacting to frustration about your ongoing health needs, realize that he or she may be feeling powerless and inadequate. (However, if your doctor's abrasiveness is a pattern, you'll need to take some action, like speaking with your doctor about the problem or changing doctors.)

- Be congenial. Don't just treat your doctor as merely a means to further tests or a new prescription. This also goes for the often overworked and harried office staff.

- Send a thank-you note if a doctor or other staff member has been especially helpful. For instance, if your doctor arranges for you to see a specialist that you requested, write and say you appreciate his or her efforts.

- Let your doctor know when a nurse or assistant has been helpful to you. It's important to commend good work.

- Come prepared for appointments by bringing notes and questions; this is especially important if you have memory problems. Yet don't overwhelm your doctor with unnecessary information or endless questions. Keep in mind that his or her time with you is limited and prioritize your concerns.

- Let your doctor know in person or in writing when you're unhappy with your care to give him or her an opportunity to respond to your concerns before you register a formal complaint.

- If you can't resolve matters, don't remain in a doctor's practice unhappily. Switch doctors.

Reminders

You're ultimately in charge of your health care. Trust your instincts regardless of what others say.

Since your disability is hidden, expect that some health care professional may dismiss your symptoms. Don't personalize their reactions.

If one doctor can't find out what's wrong, see another.

Let your doctor know verbally or in writing when you're dissatisfied. Approach him or her diplomatically, yet assertively.

Switch doctors if yours doesn't take your symptoms seriously.

Doctors don't always know best. You are capable of learning what's best for your body by listening to it.

Research all medications, vitamins, surgery, and injections before you decide to try them (whenever possible).

CHAPTER **12**

Psychotherapists: Helpful versus Unhelpful

I went to this psychologist who my friend recommended. I wanted to focus on my health problems, but he wanted to talk about my mother. He said that I wasn't getting better because I was still angry at her. It took me six months to stop seeing him because I thought that he knew best. Now I'm seeing a new therapist who truly understands about chronic illness. It's such a relief.

—Anne, age thirty-two,
living with endometriosis

Physicians try to heal your body; psychotherapists aspire to heal your mind. Seeing a trained, competent, supportive therapist can help you to accept your hidden disability, learn new ways of coping, and feel less depressed and anxious. But if your therapist isn't skilled in working with people with hidden disabilities, counseling can make you feel discouraged and inadequate. The keys to a positive experience are finding the right therapist for you and entering into treatment with realistic expectations.

When Should You Seek Help?

When Karen, age forty-seven, saw her physician for degenerative hearing loss, the doctor noticed she looked downhearted. Karen confided that wearing hearing aids and dealing with others' questions were making her depressed. She was isolating herself from others, spending too much time sleeping, overeating, and even having thoughts of suicide. Her doctor referred her to a therapist skilled in treating people with health problems.

Sheila, a thirty-nine-year-old with severe allergies, went to her doctor to find out why she had developed digestive problems. The doctor summarily dismissed her new symptoms as stress and suggested that she see a "shrink."

Karen and Sheila were beginning therapy with different expectations. Karen realized that she needed help. She was hopeful that therapy could support her in accepting the reality of her hearing loss. Sheila left her doctor's office feeling demoralized. She interpreted her doctor's comments as implying that she was neurotic and hypochondriacal. She took his referral to a therapist as a sign that she was a weak and hopeless case.

Do Karen and Sheila both need therapy? By having suicidal thoughts, Karen sounds clinically depressed. Seeking therapy may offer her tools to cope more effectively, as well as a safe place to grieve her losses.

But what about Sheila? If Sheila, like Karen, is overwhelmed by feelings of depression, anxiety, or frustration about her situation, therapy may help. But the doctor's referral without a thorough assessment of Sheila's digestive problems is questionable. Doctors are sometimes quick to assume that disorders are psychosomatic when they're stumped about a diagnosis.

For Sheila to have a positive experience in therapy, she needs to feel motivated to go, aside from her doctor's pressure. If she expects treatment to cure her stomach problems, she will likely be disappointed. Because her doctor has implied that her symptoms are all stress related, she may enter therapy feeling angry at having to come, ashamed of being perceived as deficient, or desperate to find the psychological "cure" for her health problem. These unrealistic expectations are a setup for Sheila to resent being in therapy and for therapy to fail.

Just because people in your life are doubting your symptoms doesn't mean that you need therapy. Since your disability is hidden, it's common for others to attribute your symptoms to stress. And there may be other reasons why people insist that you see a therapist. For instance, if your doctor or partner is pressuring you to go, he or she may feel unsure of how to help you. Your partner may also harbor the unrealistic expectation that a therapist will cure your health problems.

There are times, however, when it is appropriate to see a therapist. Deciding to see a therapist is not a sign that you're inadequate or that your medical problems aren't real. Being in counseling may help you manage your feelings about living with a hidden disability. A compassionate and skillful counselor can teach you new skills to cope and grow. You can also learn how to respond assertively to questions and comments from others and to stand up for your rights.

Sometimes therapy is essential. You should seek help if:

- You're depressed because of your hidden disability; this is especially important if you are having suicidal thoughts.

- You have an eating disorder, such as under- or overeating or bulimia (bingeing and purging).

- Your emotional state is making it difficult for you to perform your daily activities.

- You can't sleep because of worries or obsessive thoughts.

- Your relationships with others are being jeopardized.

- The trauma of having health problems is bringing up traumas from your past.

- You've developed unhealthy habits, such as excessive drinking or drug use.

- You're participating in self-destructive activities, such as unsafe sex.

- You're angry most of the time.

How to Find the Right Therapist

Once you've decided to seek counseling, your next challenge is to find the right therapist for you. Since you'll be sharing intimate thoughts and feelings, you'll want a therapist who is trustworthy, experienced, and sensitive. You'll also want a therapist who recognizes the difficulties of living with a hidden disability.

Most graduate schools in psychotherapy teach next to nothing about how to help clients who suffer from health problems. In fact, sometimes the training received can be counterproductive, since many traditionally trained therapists learn to attribute most problems to childhood traumas. Therefore, you'll want to make sure that your therapist has had some experience either personally or professionally with hidden disabilities.

To start your search, ask friends, co-workers, or family members for referrals (keeping in mind that just because your acquaintance liked his or her therapist, this doesn't mean you and this therapist will click). You can also get names from physicians, health organizations, support groups, therapist referral services, the newspaper, or your local phone book.

Beginning Your Search

Consider "interviewing" a therapist by phone prior to scheduling an appointment. While it may feel intimidating to ask him or her questions, remember that you are the consumer. You'll be able to get somewhat of a feel

---

Types of Psychotherapists

While each state may differ, these are generally the types of mental health professionals who practice psychotherapy:

- Psychiatrists are medical doctors who do a residency in psychiatry. They are the only mental health professionals who can prescribe drugs or order medical tests. Some psychiatrists limit their practices to prescribing medications and don't do counseling.

- Psychologists hold doctorates in psychology. In addition to offering psychotherapy, some psychologists conduct psychological testing.

- Clinical social workers have master's degrees and specialize in psychotherapy. They have had specialized training in the social roots of psychological problems.

- Marriage, family, and child counselors have master's degrees, and their training has been primarily in family-oriented perspectives. However, most counselors also do individual counseling.

- Psychiatric nurses are registered nurses with master's degrees in psychiatric nursing.

- Interns are in training. They work under the supervision of a licensed psychotherapist. They may be at an agency only temporarily.

---

for his or her personality, working style, and experience with people suffering from hidden disabilities. Most therapists should be willing to talk to you for about ten minutes. If they aren't, this may be a cue to find another therapist.

When you meet the therapist, see how comfortable you feel talking to him or her. Is he or she warm and sensitive? Does the therapist interact with you? Does he or she seem sharp and intuitive? Does the therapist accept your perspective about your health problems or do you sense some blaming or skepticism? While the first session only starts the process, you should get some idea of what it feels like being in the room with this therapist. Trust your instincts; if something doesn't feel right, consider seeking help elsewhere.

What Kind of Therapy Works Best?

Perusing the therapy ads in the phone book might feel overwhelming. One therapist touts his or her knowledge of cognitive-behavioral therapy, while another extols the virtues of depth therapy. Some advertise their knowledge of techniques you've never even heard of. How do you know what type of therapy is most effective for someone struggling with a hidden disability?

Questions to Ask Prospective Therapists

- Do you work with people short-term as well as long-term?

- How long have you been out of graduate school? Are you licensed?

- What is your theoretical orientation?

- What are your fees? (If necessary, you can ask: Do you have a sliding scale?)

- What's your policy about charging for cancellations? (Note that there are a wide range of policies from not allowing any cancellations without a penalty to a more reasonable twenty-four-hour-notice policy. Given your health problems, this may be a consideration.)

- How many people have you treated with hidden disabilities? How do you work with them?

- What do you think are the unique challenges for people whose disabilities are hidden?

- Some people believe that health problems are all caused by emotional difficulties. What do you think?

- What role, if any, do you see the past playing in current health problems?

- Do you believe that people create their health problems and that they can then cure them?

- Since people have a variety of reactions to working with someone ill or in pain, how would you know if your own personal buttons got pushed? What would you do?

- Have you had any personal experience with chronic illness or pain?

While each therapeutic style has its strengths and limitations, some are more suitable for those challenged by health problems. At the same time, the personality and talents of a particular therapist may be even more important than the type of therapy he or she practices. Also, many therapists consider themselves "eclectic," meaning that they draw from a variety of methods and techniques and aren't wedded to one approach. Such versatility may be an advantage for a person with a hidden disability who desires both practical skills for coping as well as support and comfort.

The following sections describe some of the more popular types of therapies with the potential pros and cons for someone with a hidden disability. Read through the list and see which appeal to you. There are so many varieties of therapies that it's not possible to describe them all. Carefully check out any method that you haven't heard about before. Be cautious of unorthodox, fringe approaches. Also, be wary of people who label themselves as therapists but who are not licensed or license-eligible.

Depth Therapy

There are various styles of treatment that fall under the umbrella of "depth therapy" or "insight-oriented therapy," for instance, psychodynamic, psychoanalytic, objects relations, and self psychology. Generally speaking, the therapist views problems in the present as originating in unresolved conflicts and traumas of the past. He or she uses such techniques as making interpretations, analyzing dreams, and examining your reactions to him or her (referred to as "transference"). The hope is that through developing a deep and trusting relationship with your therapist, you'll repair feelings of low self-esteem and self-hate.

Pros for People with Hidden Disabilities

This approach may be useful if childhood traumas are resurfacing and exacerbating your suffering. For instance, if your chronic pain is reminding you of years of abuse or neglect by parents, depth therapy may help you to better understand and release these feelings.

Cons for People with Hidden Disabilities

Most depth therapists recommend or even insist that you remain in therapy long-term (a couple of years or more) to accomplish your goals. Also, because your disability is hidden, some therapists may attribute your symptoms to unresolved problems of the past, which can leave you feeling blamed or criticized. Another disadvantage is that you may become insightful about your past but learn few concrete skills for daily coping.

Cognitive-Behavioral Therapy

This therapy suggests that emotional suffering results from distorted thinking. By seeing an event realistically, you'll then feel better. Also, by practicing new, healthy behavior, painful feelings are diminished. Cognitive-behavioral therapists generally focus on the present, although they'll ask about the past in order to uncover why you've developed dysfunctional behavior and negative thinking. Exercises and homework assignments teach ways to identify and modify distorted thinking.

Pros for People with Hidden Disabilities

The short-term, structured approach of cognitive-behavioral therapy has proven highly effective for anxiety disorders, chronic pain, and depression. You learn that any experience in life is manageable if you modify your negative, automatic thoughts. Clients can immediately recognize new strategies for change.

Cons for People with Hidden Disabilities

If you want a more unstructured setting to share your thoughts, feelings, and childhood memories, you may be frustrated by this task-oriented approach. Also, you'll need to be committed to practicing the exercises on your own and doing the homework.

Existential Therapy

Existential therapy presumes that emotional pain is not unique to each person because of childhood problems. Instead, it proposes that all individuals suffer due to the eventuality of death, alienation from others, and the limits of a human life. Therapists help you to realize that everyone suffers because life is finite, and guide you to find meaning within your suffering.

Pros for People with Hidden Disabilities

Developing a hidden disability can precipitate an existential crisis. You've lost the protective shield of denial, that is, the erroneous belief that illness only happens to other people. Existential therapy can allow you to draw strength from your newly acquired wisdom and to accept life as it is.

Cons for People with Hidden Disabilities

If you're not wanting to confront these ultimate truths, existential therapy can possibly increase your anxiety. Also, while you can develop a more realistic understanding of your life, you may not gain basic survival skills, such as how to assert your needs.

Spiritual/Transpersonal Therapy

Therapists practicing from this approach see people as being in a continual process of emotional and spiritual growth, and they encourage this deepening state through meditation, prayer, yoga, and other religious practices. Some may see your pain and suffering as alienation from God or another Higher Power.

Pros for People with Hidden Disabilities

If you're oriented toward a religious or spiritual perspective, you might appreciate using spirituality to cope with having a hidden disability. Illness can be viewed as an opportunity for deeper wisdom.

Cons for People with Hidden Disabilities

If you're not spiritually inclined, this approach might turn you off. Also, some practitioners might espouse New Age beliefs about illness that may offend you; for instance, a therapist might say that you've caused your disease and can cure it through positive thinking. This method also may lack the practical skills that are helpful to manage your anxiety or depression.

Group Therapy

There are numerous types of group therapy approaches, which include general therapy groups; women's or men's groups; and illness-specific support groups (e.g., chronic pain, diabetes, depression, etc.). The focus of the group may vary from long-term and in-depth support to brief and practical assistance.

Pros for People with Hidden Disabilities

If you're in a group focused on health problems, you'll meet people struggling with similar issues. Even in a more general group, you'll learn that you're not alone in having problems. You can practice communication skills in the group, such as assertiveness training, which can be applied to your daily life.

Cons for People with Hidden Disabilities

You'll need to share the hour with others and will have less time to discuss your problems than in individual therapy. In a general group, some members may not be sensitive to your disability since it's hidden (although it's possible to transform this into a "pro" by using this as an opportunity to assert yourself in a safe, controlled environment). If your group concentrates on health problems, you'll want to make sure the focus remains productive and proactive so it doesn't turn into a gripe session.

Red Flags in Therapy

You've explored different types of therapy and chosen an approach that attracts you. Perhaps you've found a therapist who makes you feel accepted, understood, and supported. Your therapist is offering you new techniques for coping, and your fear and depression have subsided.

But what if you're not comfortable with your sessions? Maybe your therapist is making comments about your hidden disability that feel insulting to you, but you're not sure how to respond. Or he or she is being overly solicitous and not respecting the client/therapist boundary. You've invested time, money, and effort into building a therapeutic relationship. What do you do next?

Being human, therapists have off days. While they attempt to be supportive and sensitive, at times they may say something that's off base or even hurts your feelings. Giving constructive feedback to your therapist will improve his or her ability to help you.

Some therapy experiences, however, do more harm than good. Perhaps your therapist believes that physical problems are all psychological, which offends you. Or maybe your therapist is struggling with his or her own emotional reactions to the difficulties you present, a phenomenon called "countertransference." One example of countertransference is when therapists become judgmental toward their clients out of anxiety about becoming ill themselves.

Let's look at some "red flags" in therapy, with suggestions of how to respond.

"Your Health Problems Are Psychological"

You've just started seeing a psychiatrist who came highly recommended. After recounting your year-long struggle with chronic neck and shoulder pain, your therapist asks you about your childhood. When you share that your father abused you, he responds, "Aha! I think we've found the answer to your pain problem. You're still carrying the weight of the abuse on your shoulders."

When you balk at this pat answer, your therapist remains adamant, and adds ominously, "Unless you heal your childhood traumas, your pain will never go away." You leave the session feeling misunderstood and anxious.

Suggestions

This therapist seems to want to sign you up for years of costly therapy. While you might vent long-buried feelings about your father, it's doubtful that you'll learn how to better cope with your pain. You should trust your instincts and find another therapist, remembering to interview prospective therapists by phone about their views on health problems.

"You've Caused Your Pain, Now Cure It"

You see an experienced psychologist after being diagnosed with irritable bowel syndrome (IBS). Since you've heard that this psychologist survived cancer, you assume she will be sympathetic, and you ask no questions by phone. After you've spent twenty minutes confiding your fears and sadness about your health, she asks, "What have you learned from being ill?"

Momentarily stunned, you mutter a few words. She continues, "Your illness is a wonderful opportunity for growth. You obviously have gotten sick in order to learn something about your life. Once you learn the lessons, you'll be cured."

You counter that having IBS isn't "wonderful." You defend yourself by listing all the positive changes you have made in your life—and still your stomach hurts. She replies, "Well, you're doing something wrong, and that's why you're not cured. We need to find out what it is." You leave the session feeling angry and blamed.

Suggestions

It's not uncommon for people to espouse New Age jargon when faced with someone with a hidden disability. By blaming you for "causing" your problems or minimizing the reality of your pain, they attempt to distance themselves from their own fears about becoming ill. Allowing yourself to be blamed in this way can result in feeling more disheartened.

Don't assume that therapists who have struggled with their own health problems will be sympathetic to yours. If they think a New Age approach about being responsible for causing illness has helped them, they may assume that this will work for everyone else. Also, if they haven't dealt with their own fear and grief about their health problems, your illness may serve as a reminder of an experience they'd rather forget. It's better to find someone more sympathetic and accepting.

When Your Therapist Has a Different Agenda

You and your partner see a marriage counselor for help with the conflicts that have started since you became ill. During the session, the counselor asks about other problem areas. You reveal that your partner has trouble getting along with your mother. The next few sessions are spent talking about their difficult relationship.

Suggestions

While you both came in for help adjusting to your health problems, the counselor has detoured. While there may be value in talking about your mother after you've worked through the impact of your illness, it is important to let your therapist know how you'd like to focus the session. If the counselor persists in talking about your mother instead, find another couples counselor.

Poor Boundaries

You see a psychologist during a particularly difficult time. Your pain is flared up, and you're despairing. You're surprised when your therapist routinely goes fifteen minutes or more over the session time, confiding that he has also struggled with health problems. Your psychologist calls you during the week to see how you are doing. When you're home ill, he sends a card. While you appreciate your therapist's concern, his actions seem excessive, even intrusive.

Suggestions

The therapeutic relationship is a unique one. You share intimate details of your life with someone who remains silent about their own. The structure of therapy—a set appointment time, a "fifty-minute hour," and the relationship's confines of the office—affords you a sense of privacy and safety. Because your therapist doesn't burden you with his problems, you don't have to take care of him. The "rules" of therapy help you feel protected.

You're right to feel uncomfortable with this therapist's violations of the boundaries of therapy. If you think that he would be responsive, you could first speak with your therapist about your concerns. However, if you feel that there's no hope, find another therapist with better boundaries.

The "Distancing" Therapist

You've seen a clinical social worker for six months and feel that she has been helpful and sympathetic. Yet during this time, your health has deteriorated, and you're depressed. During a particularly rough flare-up, your therapist reacts in ways that feel rejecting and hurtful. She is late for two appointments, raises your fee with little explanation, and has also started taking notes during your sessions without any explanation for the change in procedure. But you're reluctant to say anything for fear of alienating her further.

But when she "forgets" an appointment and leaves you sitting in the waiting room for an hour, you summon up your courage and tell her that you feel hurt. With little emotion, she says, "Maybe I'm not the right therapist for you. You don't seem to be feeling any better. Would you like a referral to another person?" You leave feeling completely abandoned.

Suggestions

What happened to make this therapist turn her back on you? Perhaps she was experiencing a countertransference response. Maybe your ongoing health crises were confronting your therapist with her own mortality and the randomness of health problems. Or she may be the type of person who gets frustrated easily when clients don't make quick progress.

You do yourself a favor by speaking with your therapist as soon as problems start. Your therapist should respect your time. She shouldn't raise your fee precipitously, with no discussion or explanation. While it can be intimidating to confront your therapist, remember that you are a consumer of her services and are entitled to respect and information.

When Therapy Makes You Feel Worse, Not Better

You're experiencing incapacitating anxiety about your hidden disability. You can't sleep and have no appetite. Every waking moment is spent preoccupied with worst-case scenarios.

During the first session with your new therapist, you recount your terror about your health problems. Your therapist suggests that you express your feelings, and you cry deeply. But you return home even more agitated.

During the next two sessions, your therapist continues to encourage you to get in touch with your feelings. She even uses exercises that intensify feelings. When you finally tell her that you're feeling worse, not better, she insists that this is normal; you should just be patient. You're not sure what to believe.

Suggestion

In theory, expressing deep feelings should lead to emotional release and relief. But this only works if you're avoiding your feelings. If, instead, you're overwhelmed by anxiety and depression, increasing the feelings can make you even more incapacitated. You need help learning to manage your emotional state. A more practical approach, like cognitive-behavioral therapy, teaches you to counteract negative thoughts that produce anxiety.

The Inflexible Therapist

You see a well-known psychologist after being diagnosed with fibromyalgia. When you speak with the therapist over the phone, he sounds experienced in helping clients with health problems. When you enter the therapist's office, you notice that the chairs are poorly designed for your bad back. You ask if you could bring in the hard-back waiting room chair. The therapist responds, "No, because I don't want to disturb the waiting room." You settle uncomfortably into a too-soft chair.

At the end of the session, the therapist goes over his policies. He doesn't allow cancellations without a seventy-two-hour notice. You inform the therapist that given your unpredictable flare-ups, you may not know three days in advance if you'll have to cancel, and ask for a twenty-four-hour arrangement. The therapist counters that there are no exceptions to this policy.

Suggestions

While this therapist claimed to be sensitive to those with disabilities, his actions contradict his words. The therapist seems oblivious to the hidden, yet real, aspects of your disability; since you look fine, he assumes that you have no special needs. The therapist's unwillingness to bring in a more suitable chair or to make allowances for your flare-ups shows that he doesn't have the flexibility to work with someone with a hidden disability. Call another therapist and ask over the phone whether the therapist can provide a suitable chair. Also, inquire in advance about cancellation policies.

The Pitying Therapist

At first, your new therapist seemed sympathetic. But as you've shared in detail your years of pain and fatigue, she seems to feel sorry for you, saying things like, "How awful! How can you tolerate such pain?" While you realize that she is trying to make you feel understood, instead you feel like a pathetic loser. After seeing your therapist, you feel truly cursed by your bad luck in developing a hidden disability.

Suggestions

Your therapist may be guarding against her own fears of illness by feeling sorry for you. Yet the therapist is doing you no favor; her pity makes you feel damaged and broken. You don't want your own therapist to convey that you're living a miserable and hopeless existence.

Your therapist needs to help you put your situation in perspective. However difficult your plight, you're not the only one struggling with chronic pain or illness. And there are many ways to manage and cope. Switch to a therapist who can both understand and impart hope.

Viewing Biochemical Problems as Strictly Psychological

You've struggled throughout your life with severe problems paying attention and concentrating. Your teachers and parents were at a loss about how to help you. Throughout your life, you've wrestled with depression and low self-esteem.

Leafing through a book on attention deficit disorder (ADD), you wonder whether this genetic disorder was the cause of your school problems and your lifelong feelings of inadequacy. You make an appointment with a counselor recommended by a close friend.

After describing your perennial struggle, your counselor zeros in on your family relationships. When you mention that your parents divorced when you were ten, he concludes that you were distracted by family problems and depressed by your father's departure. He discounts the diagnosis of adult ADD as a "fad," and suggests that you're in denial of the childhood roots of your depression.

Suggestions

This therapist has little knowledge about your disability. While some therapists doubt the existence of ADD, new scientific evidence, including specialized brain scans, suggests that there are distinct features in the brains of those with ADD. Thus, while family stressors may have played some role in your feeling depressed, the frustration of having undiagnosed and untreated ADD in and of itself can be depressing.

Your best bet is to find a therapist who specializes in ADD to diagnose and treat you. Your counselor can also help you find a physician for an evaluation of medications used to treat this problem.

Working Collaboratively with Your Therapist

Having a supportive therapist to see each week can help ease the loneliness and fear of having a hidden disability. While some counselors may be ill-equipped to help people with health problems, there are many competent and caring therapists. In addition to recognizing and responding to red flags, what else can you do to make therapy an optimal experience? The following suggestions offer ways to help therapy be a positive experience.

Have Realistic Goals

If your expectations are unrealistic, you'll be disappointed. Examples of unrealistic goals for therapy are:

- believing therapy will solve all your health problems

- expecting your therapist to always know what you need

- not working between sessions on improving your morale and creating a healthier lifestyle

- expecting to feel better right away

- believing that therapy will get at the "root cause" of your medical problems and will "cure" you once and for all

Therapy can help you cope with your pain and fatigue, but it isn't a panacea. If, for instance, you are living with chronic pain, therapy may help you manage your anxiety and lessen your muscle tension. Consequently, you may feel better. But if you come to therapy expecting to rid yourself permanently of all your medical problems, you will likely be disappointed.

While a good therapist should have some sense of how to help you, you know intuitively what's helpful. Work collaboratively with your therapist. If you're unhappy with your sessions, tell your therapist and develop a new plan of action together. (If your therapist seems threatened by your bringing up dissatisfaction, this may be a red flag to switch.)

Come Prepared to Work

You only have a finite amount of time together. Think about your sessions in between, and write any reflections or insights in a journal. Prior to the session, plan what you'd like to focus on during that time. If you depend on your therapist to shape the hour, you'll be robbed of the opportunity to use the time as you see fit.

Keep Your Appointments

While there may be emergencies when you have to cancel, whenever possible keep your appointments. Be on time. Progress can be impeded if therapy is inconsistent.

Know When It's Time to Stop

If your instincts tell you that you've gotten as much as you can from therapy, talk to your therapist about termination. You may decide to immediately stop going, set an end time a little in the future, or gradually phase out by putting more and more time between sessions.

Consider Medications

If a genuine effort at participating in therapy doesn't help your depression or anxiety, consider trying medications. There are a number of newer antidepressants [called Selective Serotonin Reuptake Inhibitors (SSRI), such as Prozac, Zoloft, and Paxil] which may have fewer side effects than older antidepressants. They can sometimes help with anxiety as well. Research the pros and cons of medication, and seek an evaluation by a psychiatrist if you're interested.

Reminders

Therapy can be a safe place to get support and learn new skills. But if something doesn't feel right, voice your concerns or change therapists.

For therapy to be effective, you must be an active partner. Use the hour productively, and think about your sessions during the week.

Being in therapy can help you to cope with your hidden disability. But be realistic—expecting therapy to cure your health problems will lead to frustration and disappointment.

You are entitled to work with a therapist who is sympathetic, knowledgeable, and supportive about your hidden disability. If your therapist believes that your health problems are all in your head, find another therapist.

Advice for Loved Ones

Everyone asks how Sarah's doing. They're really worried about her.
I feel selfish saying this, but what about me? I'm suffering, too.

—Kimberly, age thirty-one,
whose partner has Lyme's disease

A hidden disability is a family affair. When your loved one hurts, so do you. Your world is also turned upside down. You must deal with your loved one's confusion and fear while managing your own. And you have to do all of this while coping with other people's skepticism and doubt. Kimberly says:

Nothing in my life has prepared me for the overwhelming feelings caused by living with someone with a chronic illness. Sometimes I feel so scared; yet I don't want her to know. I need to be strong for her. And other times I'm angry at her. I know it doesn't make sense, but in some ways I blame her for ruining our lives. We used to have so much fun together. Now she's depressed and really suffering. Of course, I feel guilty for feeling this way. I guess the bottom line is that I feel helpless. I wish there was more I could do.

Helplessness is one of the most common feelings associated with loving someone with a hidden disability. You'd give anything to help your loved one feel better, but you don't know how. Suggestions don't work. Trying to cheer him or her up falls flat. Giving your loved one articles to read just overwhelms him or her. Sometimes all you can do is sit and listen, but this doesn't feel like nearly enough.

The first step in helping your loved one is taking care of yourself. Know that your feelings are normal and expected. You're stressed out and overwhelmed by the situation as well. Yet your feelings may be overlooked—not only by others but by yourself. You may try to be stoic and strong, like Kimberly, but inside you feel neglected and anxious. Following are some common circumstances and reactions that occur when you love someone with a hidden disability (your responses will vary according to your unique relationship with the person):

- Fears: uncertainty about your loved one's health, the future, whether your relationship will survive the strain

- Life changes: pressure to help out more; less leisure time; less money

- Instability: broken appointments; can't make plans

- Losses: grief for old relationship/the way things used to be; loss of activities you used to do together

- Frustration and anger: your fuse is shorter

- Guilt: feeling bad about being impatient or about doing things without your loved one

- Isolation: friends and family may not really understand; your loved one may become withdrawn

- Doubt from others: having to defend your loved one

- Dealing with the medical system: financial and emotional strain

- Children: worrying about the kids; having to become more responsible for them

- Your own doubt: wondering whether your loved one is exaggerating his or her symptoms

Can you relate to these reactions? It's common to be faced with a myriad of emotions when your loved one develops a hidden disability. Your feelings parallel your loved one's: grief, anger, depression, fear. Yet, as Kimberly noted, others may not recognize your suffering. While friends ask how your loved one is doing, they may overlook your pain. You may resent all the attention he or she receives from friends, doctors, and therapists. You may feel neglected, especially since you're giving more than you're receiving. Then you feel guilty and selfish for resenting your loved one.

You're also confronted with others who are dubious about hidden disabilities. Having to defend your loved one is awkward and uncomfortable. For instance, Kimberly recalled a difficult conversation with her mother:

My mother called and asked how Sarah was doing. When I told her that she was having joint pain, my mother said that maybe a lot of her pain was due to stress. She thought Sarah might get better if she weren't so high strung. I was really annoyed, but I was at a loss for words. I didn't want to get angry at my mother, but I also didn't want Sarah's illness to be demeaned.

You also may be confused about how to respond to the doubts of others. You want to advocate for your loved one, but you also don't want to make a scene or alienate yourself from others. Or perhaps you have some doubts yourself about your loved one's symptoms. Do you sometimes wonder whether he or she is exaggerating? Or do you speculate that some of his or her pain may be caused by depression?

Having doubts is understandable since your loved one's disability is hidden. But harboring suspicion can drive a wedge in your relationship. To preserve your relationship, you need to be supportive of your loved one. It helps to learn as much as you can about hidden disabilities, such as by reading this book, searching the Internet, and occasionally going along for doctor visits.

Your love and compassion are essential in helping your loved one live well with a hidden disability. You don't have to do anything special; simply listening to him or her and being present are healing acts. Like Kimberly, you may feel like listening isn't enough and wish you could do more. While you'd love to alleviate his or her physical burden, this isn't always possible. But remaining committed to your relationship will make his or her emotional pain more tolerable.

You can also ask your loved one what he or she needs. Don't assume that you should know. The meaning of support differs for each person. The very act of asking how you could be supportive is supportive; it also communicates caring and concern. Here are some other ways to help your loved one and yourself:

Do:

- Take breaks for yourself.

- Know the signs of burnout (see below).

- Consider taking a planned vacation alone or with a friend.

- Join with others. For instance, attend your loved one's support group. Contact the organization Well Spouse (see appendix D).

- Continue your enjoyed activities even if you do them alone or with others.

- Believe in your loved one: Even if his or her disability is hidden, it's still real.

- Seek counseling for yourself if you become depressed; consider counseling together if there's strain.

- Go out with friends and family regularly.

- Exercise—even short walks can help relieve tension and stress.
- Set limits with your loved one when necessary, especially if he or she is obsessing.
- Offer help with concrete tasks, such as shopping and cooking.
- Remind him or her of your love and commitment.

Don't:

- Blame yourself for not doing more.
- Feel guilty for having your own life.
- Give up your own needs and interests.
- Overwhelm your loved one with suggestions and advice.
- Take your frustration out on your loved one.
- Try to cheer him or her up if this isn't helpful.
- Blame him or her for becoming ill.
- Offer explanations for his or her hidden disability, for instance, "bad karma."

Signs of Burnout

Here are some signs that you may be overloaded in dealing with your loved one's hidden disability. While trying our suggestions may help, you may need to take a few days or weeks away from your loved one. A support group or counseling can also help. Check all that apply:

_____ feeling exhausted

_____ catching colds easily

_____ gaining or losing weight

_____ becoming sedentary

_____ having panic attacks

_____ experiencing insomnia

_____ having problems over- or undereating

_____ using drugs or alcohol

_____ eating too much junk food

_____ feeling hopeless or despairing

_____ crying easily

_____ avoiding your loved one

_____ becoming easily frustrated with your loved one or with others

_____ considering ending the relationship or friendship

Reminders

A hidden disability turns your world upside down, too.

It's normal to feel a myriad of emotions, including helplessness, sadness, frustration, anxiety, and guilt.

While you cannot eliminate your loved one's disability, your love and support are enormously helpful. Just listening to your loved one offers comfort and solace.

Take care of yourself: exercise, connect with others, take time to yourself.

Seek counseling if you need added support, especially if you're depressed.

Advice for Psychotherapists

As a therapist, you've likely received no training on how to work effectively with clients who have hidden disabilities. Continuing education classes on this subject are hard to find. Yet more and more people are succumbing to puzzling symptoms: immune disorders; psychiatric disabilities, such as attention deficit disorders; and chronic pain. These clients come into therapy feeling defeated, hypersensitive to criticism, and angry.

Consequently, they're challenging clients. Given that you enjoy seeing clients improve, hidden disability sufferers can frustrate you. Their symptoms often persist in spite of your best efforts. The usual techniques of insight and interpretation may not alleviate their emotional and physical pain. During relapses, they become depressed, maybe even suicidal. Given that health problems are a high-risk factor for suicide, you often have to add crisis appointments and seek consultation.

Clients often come to you with unrealistic expectations. They've been dismissed by medical professionals who either can't find a physical basis for their problem or have exhausted their ability to help. Sometimes clients are told outright that their hidden disability is "all in their head." They then expect therapy to cure their pain. When therapy doesn't eliminate symptoms, clients feel even more frustrated and despairing. Those with psychiatric diagnoses, like bipolar disorder or obsessive-compulsive disorder, may have tried therapy before with little success. Exploration of the past hasn't ameliorated their symptoms. Given the stigma of a psychiatric problem, they generally arrive in your office feeling ashamed and weak.

It's natural to experience strong emotions when working with these clients. Here are a few of the most common ones:

- Frustration: While you're trying your hardest, the client remains depressed.

- Anxious: You worry whether your client's plight could happen to you or someone you love. You're anxious that the client may become completely incapacitated and seriously consider suicide. If you've experienced medical problems yourself, you may become flooded by unpleasant memories.

- Doubt: You wonder whether his or her symptoms are psychosomatic.

- Sadness: You're saddened by your client's considerable pain and suffering.

- Helplessness: You wish there was more you could do.

- Anger: You're angry when your client is needy yet resistant to your suggestions.

- Overwhelmed: The client's insatiable needs leave you feeling inadequate and overwhelmed.

Seeing a client ill and in pain can evoke an array of feelings in you. Your feelings may parallel your client's view. Just as your client feels anxious about the future, you also worry about his or her well-being. Your client's anger at the world may make you angry at him or her for being so negative and critical. Your client questions the validity of his or her symptoms, as you do. Given your strong emotional reaction, it can be hard to maintain a therapeutic distance.

Having strong responses may not harm your client. It all depends on what you do with them. Frustration, for instance, can be manifested in various ways. You might become impatient with your client and admonish him or her for not doing relaxation exercises. If you're anxious, you might distance yourself from your client's pain, leaving him or her feeling alone and abandoned. But countertransference can also be used to help guide your client. The key is being aware of your own material; know what's emerging inside of you.

Here are some common countertransference reactions to working with clients with hidden disabilities:

- Distancing: Overwhelmed by your client's suffering, you detach from him or her emotionally. Or, while working with a client who has a psychiatric disorder, you're uncomfortable being in the room with him or her. Common examples of distancing: starting sessions late, feeling bored and sleepy, daydreaming, breaking appointments, and/or taking copious notes during the session.

- Criticizing: You're frustrated by your client's slow progress and scold him or her for not doing more.

- Maintaining poor boundaries: You bind feelings of helplessness by violating boundaries. Examples: calling your client at home, going over time, offering extremely low-fee or free sessions.

- Rejecting: You unconsciously wish your client would terminate sessions. You raise the fee, change the appointment time, or appear cold and unapproachable.

- Being impatient: You're irritable and edgy.

- Obsessing: Your countertransference is so overpowering that you think about your client night and day.

- Being skeptical: You don't believe your client's version of his or her symptoms and attribute psychological origins.

Consider the following example: A psychologist saw a thirty-five-year-old woman, Kirsten, with lupus. Kirsten began therapy after a month-long hospital stay where her lungs and kidneys failed. The client was overcome with fear about having a reoccurrence. She also worried about the impact of her illness on her five-year-old daughter.

After a few weeks of therapy, the therapist noticed that he'd become increasingly more distracted during sessions. While the client cried, he'd daydream about grocery shopping. The psychologist started dreading seeing this client, even though Kirsten was a thoughtful and likable person. When he "forgot" about a session, he realized that he needed consultation.

In consultation, he admitted that his worst fear was developing a serious illness. He also feared his wife's becoming disabled. The suddenness of Kirsten's disease was particularly unsettling. The therapist realized that he was distancing himself from his client to avoid dealing with his own issues about illness.

He used his insight to try to create a therapeutic bond. He told her:

> First, I want to apologize to you for missing our session. I want to let you know, too, that I've been thinking a lot about what happened and about our relationship. I've been noticing that when you talk about your illness, I sometimes detach; I go somewhere else. I've tried to figure out why. I think part of it is my own anxiety about illness. It also makes me feel sad that you have lupus. I wish that there was more that I could do. But I realize that what I *can* do is to be here for you as best as I can.

Kirsten was disarmed by her therapist's self-disclosure. Given that she had noticed his distancing, she was relieved and touched by his honesty. She began talking about how other people also move away from her, and how hard that is. She appreciated his efforts to remain connected.

The key, then, is to become aware of your own reaction and channel it in therapeutic ways. Your countertransference helps you to experience what your client feels. If you feel anxious, you're likely in touch with his or her considerable anxiety. Your feelings can be used as a bridge to make your client feel less alone.

Here are some other suggestions:

- Be eclectic: Avoid being wedded to a particular technique. The psycho-analytic blank screen approach is counterproductive; clients feel isolated and need human contact and warmth.

- Be flexible: A rigid seventy-two-hour cancellation policy is unrealistic for clients with health problems.

- Be genuine: If you've made a mistake, admit it. It's okay to say, "Last week you looked overwhelmed when I inundated you with suggestions. Sometimes I feel helpless because I want you to feel better. Maybe I'm also picking up on your feelings of being helpless."

- Be realistic: Chronic illnesses are just that—chronic. Your clients will experience good and bad days. Try not to become discouraged when they have flare-ups and bouts of depression.

- Instill hope: It's easy to absorb clients' frustration and discouragement. But having two deflated people in the room isn't helpful. While the client may not be cured physically, you can help him or her restore emotional well-being.

- Believe your client: Your client has been questioned and doubted by others; he or she needs you to acknowledge his or her pain as real. The client with a psychiatric disability, for example, needs his or her disorder validated as real. Since many psychiatric problems are now believed to be genetically based, it's important for clients to know that their illness is a real, biochemical, disorder.

- Be practical: Offer concrete help such as relaxation exercises, hypnosis, guided imagery, and referrals to support groups.

- Work collaboratively: Don't assume that you know what works best for the client. It's empowering for him or her to help direct the therapy.

- Blend in cognitive-behavioral techniques: Studies show that cognitive-behavioral therapy is effective for chronic pain and illness. Depth therapy offers the client insights but neglects to teach him or her how to cope daily with self-defeating thoughts, passivity, and anxiety.

- Consider seeing family members: The family may be helping or hurting your client. A session or two with others enlists them as part of the helping team.

- Educate yourself: Learn as much as you can about your client's health problems and about the challenges of hidden disabilities.

- Seek consultation or therapy: Address your personal issues about illness and pain.

Myths and Realities about Hidden Disabilities

Myth: Chronic illness and pain are caused by unconscious memories and repressed emotions.

Reality: There are no easy answers about why people become ill. It's much more helpful to teach clients to cope than to search for the underlying causes.

Myth: If the client resolves childhood trauma, his or her health problems would be healed.

Reality: The past may have little to do with why your client has developed a hidden disability. It's more skillful to focus on the present.

Myth: The client is depressed; that's why he or she has developed chronic pain.

Reality: While some clients have a history of depression, most likely it's the hidden disability that's causing depression.

Myth: Clients cause their problems through negative thinking and stress.

Reality: Illness and pain can happen to anyone at any time. Avoid blaming the client.

Myth: Psychiatric disabilities are caused by poor parenting and early childhood traumas. Long-term psychodynamic psychotherapy is necessary.

Reality: Scientists now believe that there is a biological basis for most psychiatric disorders. Studies show that cognitive-behavioral therapy, coupled with medication when necessary, is highly effective for chronic pain and illness.

APPENDIX C

Recommended Reading

Anger

Thomas, Sandra, and Cheryl Jefferson. 1996. *Use Your Anger.* New York: Pocket Books.

Anxiety

Bourne, Edmund. 1995. *The Anxiety and Phobia Workbook,* 2d Edition. Oakland, Calif.: New Harbinger Publications.

Peurifoy, Reneau. 1995. *Anxiety, Phobias and Panic.* New York: Warner Books.

Assertiveness

Butler, Pamela. 1992. *Self-Assertion for Women.* San Francisco: HarperSanFrancisco.

Depression

Burns, David. 1980. *Feeling Good.* New York: New American Library.

Copeland, Mary Ellen. 1992. *The Depression Workbook: A Guide for Living with Depression.* Oakland, Calif.: New Harbinger Publications.

Chemicals and Toxins

Radetsky, Peter. 1997. *Allergic to the Twentieth Century*. Boston: Little, Brown & Company.

Elkington, John, et al. 1990. *The Green Consumer*. New York: Penguin Books.

Lawson, Joan. 1993. *Staying Well in a Toxic World*. Chicago: Noble Press.

Steinman, David. 1990. *Diet for a Poisoned Planet*. New York: Ballantine Books.

Employment

Repa, Barbara. 1996. *Your Rights in the Workplace*. Berkeley, Calif.: Nolo Press.

Health

Barasch, Marc. 1993. *The Healing Path*. New York: Jeremy P. Tarcher/Putnam Books.

Berkow, Robert, ed. 1997. *Merck Manual* (Home Edition). West Point: Merck & Co.

Donoghue, Paul, and Mary Siegel. 1992. *Sick and Tired of Feeling Sick and Tired*. New York: W. W. Norton.

Giller, Robert, and Kathy Matthews. 1994. *Natural Prescriptions*. New York: Ballantine Books.

Hanner, Linda, et al. 1991. *When You're Sick and Don't Know Why*. Minneapolis, Minn.: DCI Publishing.

Heiss, Gayle. 1997. *Finding the Way Home*. Fort Bragg, Calif.: QED Press.

Mindell, Earl. 1991. *Vitamin Bible*. New York: Warner Books.

Pitzele, Sefra. 1986. *We Are Not Alone*. New York: Workman Publishing.

Pollin, Irene. 1994. *Taking Charge*. New York: Times Books.

Sifton, David, ed. 1993. *The PDR Family Guide to Prescription Drugs*. Montvale: Medical Economics Data, Inc.

Somerville, Robert, ed. l996. *The Medical Advisor: The Complete Guide to Alternative and Conventional Treatments*. Richmond, Va.: Time Life.

Topf, Linda. 1995. *You Are Not Your Illness*. New York: Fireside.

Inspiration

Bosco, Antoinette. 1995. *Finding Peace Through Pain*. New York: Ballantine Books.

Chodron, Pema. 1997. *When Things Fall Apart.* Boston: Shambhala Publications.

Fabry, Joseph. 1988. *Guideposts to Meaning.* Oakland, Calif.: New Harbinger Publications.

Frankl, Viktor. 1963. *Man's Search for Meaning.* New York: Washington Square Press.

Harrison, Gavin. 1994. *In the Lap of the Buddha.* Boston: Shambhala Publications..

Kushner, Harold. 1990. *When Bad Things Happen to Good People.* New York: Random House.

Levine Stephen. 1997. *Healing into Life and Death.* New York: Doubleday.

Mitchell, Stephen. 1993. *A Book of Psalms.* New York: HarperCollins.

Mother Teresa. 1997. *In My Own Words.* New York: Random House.

Remen, Rachel Naomi. 1996. *Kitchen Table Wisdom.* New York: Riverside.

Young-Eisendrath, Polly. 1996. *The Resilient Spirit.* Reading, Mass.: Addison-Wesley.

Pain Control

Catalano, Ellen, and Kimeron Hardin. 1996. *The Chronic Pain Control Workbook.* 2d Edition. Oakland, Calif.: New Harbinger Publications.

Marcus, Norman, and Jean Arbeiter. 1995. *Freedom from Pain.* New York: Simon & Schuster.

Sternbach, Richard. 1988. *Mastering Pain.* New York: Ballantine Books.

Stress Management

Kabat-Zinn, Jon. 1990. *Full Catastrophe Living.* New York: Delacorte Press.

Davis, Martha, et al. 1995. *The Relaxation and Stress Management Workbook.* 4th Edition. Oakland, Calif.: New Harbinger Publications.

APPENDIX D

Organizations and Catalogues

Acoustic Neuroma Association
P.O. Box 12402, Atlanta, GA 30355
Tel: 404-237-8023; E-Mail: anausa@aol.com

American Academy of Allergy, Asthma and Immunology
611 E. Wells St., Milwaukee, WI 53202
1-800-822-2762; 414-272-6071; Website: www.aaaai.org

American Cancer Society
1599 Clifton Road, NE, Atlanta, GA 30329
1-800-227-2345; Website: www.cancer.org

American Chronic Pain Association
P.O. Box 850, Rocklin, CA 95677
Tel: 916-632-0922; E-Mail: acpa@ix.netcom.com

American Diabetes Association
P.O. Box 25757, 1660 Duke Street, Alexandria, VA 22314
1-800-232-3472; Website: www.diabetes.org

American Heart Association
7272 Greenville Avenue, Dallas, TX 75231
1-800-242-1793; 1-800-AHA-USA1;
Website: www.americanheart.org; E-Mail: inquire@heart.org

American Liver Foundation
1425 Pompton Avenue, Cedar Grove, NJ 07009
1-800-223-0179; Tel: 201-256-2550; Fax: 973-256-3214
Website: www.liverfoundation.org; E-Mail: info@liverfoundation.org

American Tinnitus Association
P.O. Box 5, Portland, OR 97207-0005
1-800-634-8978; Tel: 503-248-9985; Fax: 503-248-0024
Website: www.ata.org; E-Mail: tinnitus@ata.org

Arthritis Foundation
1330 West Peachtree Street; Atlanta, GA 30309
1-800-283-7800; Fax: 404-872-8694
Website: www.arthritis.org; E-Mail: help@arthritis.org

Association for Repetitive Motion Syndromes (ARMS)
P.O. Box 471973, Aurora, CO 80047 Tel: 303-369-0803

Attention Deficit Disorder Association
P.O. Box 972, Mentor, OH 44061 Tel: 216-350-9595; Website: www.add.org

CDC National Prevention Information Network [AIDS Information]
P.O. Box 6003, Rockville, MD 20849-6003 1-800-458-5231; Fax: 1-888-282-7681
Website: http://www.cdcnpin.org; E-Mail: info@cdcnpin.org

CFIDS Association
P.O. Box 220398, Charlotte, NC 28222-0398
1-800-442-3437; Fax: 704-365-9755
Website: www.cfids.org; E-Mail: info@cfids.org

Chemical Injury Information Network
P.O. Box 301, White Sulphur Springs, MT 59645-0301
Tel: 406-547-2255; Fax: 406-547-2455
Website: http://biz.comm.com/CIIN

Children and Adults with Attention Deficit Disorder (CHADD)
499 Northwest 70th Avenue, Suite 101, Plantation, FL 33317
1-800-233-4050; Website: www.chadd.org

Crohn's and Colitis Foundation
386 Park Avenue South, New York, NY 10016
1-800-932-2423 x257; Tel: 212-685-3440; Fax: 212-779-4098
Website: www.ccfa.org; E-Mail: inso@ccfa.org

Endometriosis Association International Headquarters
8585 N. 76th Place, Milwaukee, WI 53223

1-800-992-3636; Tel: 414-355-2200; Fax: 414-355-6065
Website: http://www.endometriosisassn.org; E-Mail: endo@endometriosassn.org

Epilepsy Foundation of America
4351 Garden City Drive, Landover, MD 20785
1-800-333-1000; Tel: 301-459-3700
Website: www.efa.org; E-Mail: postmaster@efa.org

Fibromyalgia Network
P.O. Box 3170, Tucson, AZ 85751-1750
1-800-523-2929; Tel: 520-290-5508; Fax: 520-290-5550
Website: www.fmnetnews.com

Hyperacusis Network
444 Edgewood Drive, Green Bay, Wisconsin 54302
902-468-4667; Fax: 920-468-0168; E-Mail: hypacusis@netnet.net

Job Accommodation Network
1-800-526-7234

Lupus Foundation of America
1300 Piccard Drive #200, Rockville, MD 20850
1-800-558-0121; Tel: 301-670-9292; Fax: 301-670-9486 Website: www.lupus.org

Lyme Disease Foundation
1 Financial Plaza, Hartford, CT 06103
1-800-886-LYME; Tel: 860-525-2000; Fax: 860-525-8425
Website: www.lyme.org; E-Mail: lymefnd@aol.com

National Alliance for the Mentally Ill
200 N. Glebe Road, Suite 1015, Arlington, VA 22203-3754
1-800-950-6264; Website: www.nami.org; E-Mail: namiofc@aol.com

National Chronic Pain Outreach Association
7979 Old Georgetown Road, Suite 100, Bethesda, MD 20814
Tel. 301-652-4948; E-Mail: mcp04@aol.com

National Depressive and Manic-Depressive Association
730 N. Franklin Street, Suite 501, Chicago, IL 60610-3526
1-800-826-3632; Fax: 312-642-7243
Website: www.ndma.org; E-Mail: myrtis@aol.com

National Digestive Diseases Information Clearinghouse
Two Information Way, Bethesda, MD 20892-3570 Tel: 301-654-3810

National Headache Foundation
428 W. St. James Place, Chicago, IL 60614
1-800-843-2256; Fax: 773-525-7357; Website: www.headaches.org

National Kidney Foundation
30 East 33rd Street, Suite 1100, New York, NY 10016
1-800-622-9010; Website: www.kidney.org

National Multiple Sclerosis Society
733 Third Avenue, 6th Floor, New York, NY 10017-3288
1-800-344-4867; Tel: 212-986-3240; Fax: 212-986-7981
Website: www.nmss.org; E-Mail: info@nmss.org

National Psoriasis Foundation
6600 SW 92nd Avenue, Suite 300, Portland, OR 97223-7195
1-800-723-9166; Website: www.psoriasis.org/npf.html
E-Mail: 76135.2746.compuserve.com

National Rosacea Society
800 South Northwest Highway, Suite 200, Barrington, IL 60010
Tel: 847-382-8971; Fax: 847-382-5567; Website: www.rosacea.org

Obsessive-Compulsive Foundation
P.O. Box 70, Milford, CT 06460-0070 Tel: 203-878-5669; Fax: 203-874-2826
Website: http://pages.prodigy.com/alwillen/ocf.html; E-Mail: jphs28a@Prodigy.com

Regional Disability and Business Technical Assistance Center
[Information on the Americans with Disabilities Act]
1-800-949-4232; Website: www.icdi.wvu.edu/tech/

Sickle Cell Disease Association of America
200 Corporate Pointe, Suite 495, Culver City, CA 90230-7633
1-800-421-8453

Thyroid Foundation of America
Ruth Sleeper Hall—RSL350, 40 Parkman Street, Boston, MA 02114
1-800-832-8321; Tel: 617-726-8500; Fax: 617-726-4136
Website: www.tsaweb.org/pub/tsa; E-Mail: tsa@clark.net

TMJ & Stress Center
P.O. Box 803394, Dallas, TX 75380
1-800-533-5121; Tel: 972-416-7676

The Well Spouse Foundation
610 Lexington Avenue, Suite 208, New York, NY 10022
1-800-838-0879; Tel: 212-644-1241; Fax: 212-644-1338
Website: www.wellspouse.org; E-Mail: wellspouse@aol.com

Catalogues of Healthy Products

Harmony Catalogue
1-800-869-3446

Seventh Generation
1-800-456-1177

Janice Corporation
1-800-JANICES

References

Chapter 1

Angelou, Maya. 1997. *I Know Why the Caged Bird Sings.* New York: Bantam.

Cantor, Carla. 1996. *Phantom Illness.* Boston: Houghton Mifflin.

Carson, Rachel. 1994. *Silent Spring.* New York: Houghton Mifflin.

Elkington, John, et al. 1990. *The Green Consumer.* New York: Penguin Books.

Frankl, Viktor. 1992. *Man's Search for Meaning.* Boston: Beacon Press.

Hanner, Linda, et al. 1991. *When You're Sick and Don't Know Why.* Minneapolis: DCI Publishing.

Johnson, Hillary. 1996. *Osler's Web.* New York: Crown Publishers.

Khalsa, Karta. l998. "When Everything Hurts." *Yoga Journal,* July/August, 48–61.

Kushner, Harold. 1990. *When Bad Things Happen to Good People.* New York: Random House.

Lawson, Joan. 1993. *Staying Well in a Toxic World.* Chicago: Noble Press.

Myss, Caroline, and Norman Sheahy. 1993. *The Creation of Health.* New York: Crown.

Radetsky, Peter. 1997. *Allergic to the Twentieth Century.* Boston: Little, Brown and Company.

Sarno, John. 1991. *Healing Back Pain.* New York: Warner Books.

Siegel, Bernie. 1986. *Love, Medicine and Miracles.* New York: Harper & Row.

Steinman, David. 1990. *Diet for a Poisoned Planet.* New York: Ballantine Books.

Taylor, Robert. 1982. *Mind or Body.* New York: McGraw-Hill.

Wittenberg, Janice. 1996. *The Rebellious Body.* New York: Insight Books.

Wolkomir, Richard. 1994. "When the Work You Do Ends Up Costing You an Arm and a Leg." *Smithsonian,* June, 90–99.

Chapter 2

American Psychiatric Association. 1994. *Diagnostic Criteria for the DSM-IV*. Washington, D.C.: American Psychiatric Association.

Kubler-Ross, Elisabeth. 1997. *On Death and Dying*. New York: Simon & Schuster.

Siegman, Aaron, et al. 1990. "The Angry Voice." *Psychosomatic Medicine*. 52: 631-643.

Spiegel, David, et al. 1989. "Effects of Psychosocial Treatment on Survival of Patients with Metastatic Breast Cancer." *The Lancet*. 2:888-891.

Chapter 3

Peck, M. Scott. 1997. *The Road Less Traveled*. New York: Simon & Schuster.

Chapter 4

Gray, John. 1992. *Men Are from Mars, Women Are from Venus*. New York: HarperCollins.

Pitzele, Sefra. 1986. *We Are Not Alone*. New York: Workman Publishing.

Chapter 7

Repa, Barbara. 1996. *Your Rights in the Workplace*. Berkeley, Calif.: Nolo Press.

Chapter 8

Elliot, Timothy, et al. "Negotiating Reality after Physical Loss: Hope, Depression, and Disability." *Journal of Personality and Social Psychology* 61:4.

Goleman, Daniel. 1995. *Emotional Intelligence*. New York: Bantam Books.

Chapter 9

Dossey, Larry. 1993. *Prayer Is Good Medicine*. San Francisco: HarperSanFrancisco.

Frankl, Viktor. 1992. *Man's Search for Meaning*. Boston: Beacon Press.

Harte, John, et. al. 1991. *Toxics A to Z*. Berkeley, California: University of California Press.

Kushner, Harold. 1990. *When Bad Things Happen to Good People*. New York: Random House.

Levine, Stephen. 1997. *Healing into Life and Death*. New York: Anchor Press/Doubleday.

Mother Teresa. 1990. "Compassion in Action." In *For the Love of God*, edited by Benjamin Shield and Richard Carlson. New York: New World Library.

Trungpa, Chogyam. 1984. *Shambhala: The Sacred Path of the Warrior*. Boulder: Shambhala. New York: Washington Square Press.

Chapter 10

Marcus, Norman, and Jean Arbeiter. 1995. *Freedom from Pain*. New York: Simon & Schuster.

Index

A

acceptance, 43-46; impact of others on, 45; self-evaluation of, 43-44; tools for cultivating, 45-46

acetaminophen, 212

adolescents. *See* teenagers

affirmations, 226-227

agoraphobia, 52

AIDS, 12, 63-64

all-or-nothing thinking, 163

altruism, 196-197

American Psychiatric Association, 38

Americans with Disabilities Act (ADA), 144-145, 152

amyotrophic lateral sclerosis (ALS), 21

anger, 32-37; hostility vs., 33-34; passive-aggressiveness as, 34; productive vs. unproductive, 35; recommended reading on, 279; related to parenting, 95-96; self-directed, 36-37; self-evaluation of, 33; techniques for managing, 34-37, 96

antidepressants, 54

anxiety, 51-54; disorders related to, 52; recommended reading on, 279; related to parenting, 94-95; techniques for managing, 53-54, 95. *See also* fears

appreciation and gratitude, 200-202

assertiveness, 171-175; barriers to, 173-174; methods of, 174-175; myths and realities about, 174; recommended reading on, 279; self-evaluation of, 171-173

associations related to hidden disabilities, 283-286

assumptions: avoiding, 59; false, 236-237

attention deficit disorder (ADD), 263

autogenics, 224-225

awareness, expanding, 55

B

babies: effects of your hidden disability on, 97-98. *See also* children

bargaining stage, 37-38

battling guilt, 58

blood pressure, 34

body, 183-194; exercise and, 189-190; fears related to, 49; healthy eating and, 190-192; making peace with your own, 185-186; reducing chemical exposure to, 192-194; self-care guidelines for, 187-192; tuning in to your own, 186-187. *See also* spirit

books, recommended for further reading, 279-286

More New Harbinger Titles

THE CHRONIC PAIN CONTROL WORKBOOK

A team of specialists in all areas of pain management detail the treatment strategies for managing and recovering from chronic pain.   *Item PN2 $17.95*

WINNING AGAINST RELAPSE

A structured program teaches you how to monitor symptoms and respond to them in a way that reduces or eliminates the possibility of relapse.   *Item WIN $14.95*

FIBROMYALGIA & CHRONIC MYOFASCIAL PAIN SYNDROME

This survival manual is the first comprehensive patient guide for managing these conditions. Readers learn how to identify trigger points, cope with chronic pain and sleep problems, and deal with the numbing effects of "fibrofog."   *Item FMS $19.95*

OVERCOMING REPITITVE MOTION INJURIES THE ROSSITER WAY

This system of partner stretches has offered immediate and lasting pain relief to thousands of workers suffering from carpal tunnel syndrome and other repetitive motion injuries and from everyday aches and pain.   *Item ROSS $15.95*

THE HEADACHE AND NECK PAIN WORKBOOK

Combines the latest research with proven alternative therapies to help sufferers of head and neck pain understand and master their condition.   *Item NECK $14.95*

CONQUERING CARPAL TUNNEL SYNDROME

Guided by symptom charts, you select the best exercises for restoring the range of motion to overworked hands and arms.   *Item CARP $17.95*

Call **toll-free 1-800-748-6273** to order. Have your Visa or Mastercard number ready. Or send a check for the titles you want to New Harbinger Publications, 5674 Shattuck Avenue, Oakland, CA 94609. Include $3.80 for the first book and 75¢ for each additional book to cover shipping and handling. (California residents please include appropriate sales tax.) Allow four to six weeks for delivery.

Prices subject to change without notice.

Some Other New Harbinger Self-Help Titles